Cutaneous Manifestations of Internal Disease

Guest Editor

NEIL S. SADICK, MD

MEDICAL CLINICS
OF NORTH AMERICA

www.medical.theclinics.com

November 2009 • Volume 93 • Number 6

SAUNDERS an imprint of ELSEVIER, Inc.

W.B. SAUNDERS COMPANY
A Division of Elsevier Inc.

1600 John F. Kennedy Boulevard ● Suite 1800 ● Philadelphia, Pennsylvania 19103-2899

http://www.theclinics.com

MEDICAL CLINICS OF NORTH AMERICA Volume 93, Number 6
November 2009 ISSN 0025-7125, ISBN-13: 978-1-4377-1241-4, ISBN-10: 1-4377-1241-X

Editor: Rachel Glover
Developmental Editor: Donald Mumford

Medical Clinics of North America (ISSN 0025-7125) is published bimonthly by Elsevier Inc., 360 Park Avenue South, New York, NY 10010-1710. Months of issue are January, March, May, July, September, and November. Periodicals postage paid at New York, NY, and additional mailing offices. Subscription prices are USD 204 per year for US individuals, USD 361 per year for US institutions, USD 105 per year for US students, USD 259 per year for Canadian individuals, USD 469 per year for Canadian institutions, USD 165 per year for Canadian students, USD 314 per year for international individuals, USD 469 per year for international institutions and USD 165 per year for international students. To receive student/resident rate, orders must be accompanied by name of affiliated institution, date of term, and the *signature* of program/residency coordinator on institution letterhead. Orders will be billed at individual rate until proof of status is received. Foreign air speed delivery is included in all *Clinics* subscription prices. All prices are subject to change without notice. **POSTMASTER:** Send address changes to *Medical Clinics of North America*, Elsevier Health Sciences Division, Subscription Customer Service, 3251 Riverport Lane, Maryland Heights, MO 63043. **Customer Service: Telephone: 1-800-654-2452** (U.S. and Canada); **1-314-447-8871** (outside U.S. and Canada). **Fax: 1-314-447-8029. E-mail: journalscustomerservice-usa@elsevier.com** (for print support); **journalsonlinesupport-usa@ elsevier.com** (for online support).

Reprints. For copies of 100 or more of articles in this publication, please contact the Commercial Reprints Department, Elsevier Inc., 360 Park Avenue South, New York, NY 10010-1710. Tel.: 212-633-3812; Fax: 212-462-1935; E-mail: reprints@elsevier.com.

Medical Clinics of North America is also published in Spanish by McGraw-Hill Interamericana Editores S. A., P.O. Box 5-237, 06500 Mexico, D.F., Mexico.

Medical Clinics of North America is covered in *MEDLINE/PubMed (Index Medicus), Current Contents, ASCA, Excerpta Medica, Science Citation Index,* and *ISI/BIOMED.*

Printed in the United States of America.

GOAL STATEMENT

The goal of *Medical Clinics of North America* is to keep practicing physicians up to date with current clinical practice by providing timely articles reviewing the state of the art in patient care.

ACCREDITATION

The *Medical Clinics of North America* is planned and implemented in accordance with the Essential Areas and Policies of the Accreditation Council for Continuing Medical Education (ACCME) through the joint sponsorship of the University of Virginia School of Medicine and Elsevier. The University of Virginia School of Medicine is accredited by the ACCME to provide continuing medical education for physicians.

The University of Virginia School of Medicine designates this educational activity for a maximum of 15 *AMA PRA Category 1 Credits*™ for each issue, 90 credits per year. Physicians should only claim credit commensurate with the extent of their participation in the activity.

The American Medical Association has determined that physicians not licensed in the US who participate in this CME activity are eligible for a maximum of 15 *AMA PRA Category 1 Credits*™ for each issue, 90 credits per year.

Credit can be earned by reading the text material, taking the CME examination online at http://www.theclinics.com/home/cme, and completing the evaluation. After taking the test, you will be required to review any and all incorrect answers. Following completion of the test and evaluation, your credit will be awarded and you may print your certificate.

FACULTY DISCLOSURE/CONFLICT OF INTEREST

The University of Virginia School of Medicine, as an ACCME accredited provider, endorses and strives to comply with the Accreditation Council for Continuing Medical Education (ACCME) Standards of Commercial Support, Commonwealth of Virginia statutes, University of Virginia policies and procedures, and associated federal and private regulations and guidelines on the need for disclosure and monitoring of proprietary and financial interests that may affect the scientific integrity and balance of content delivered in continuing medical education activities under our auspices.

The University of Virginia School of Medicine requires that all CME activities accredited through this institution be developed independently and be scientifically rigorous, balanced and objective in the presentation/discussion of its content, theories and practices.

All authors/editors participating in an accredited CME activity are expected to disclose to the readers relevant financial relationships with commercial entities occurring within the past 12 months (such as grants or research support, employee, consultant, stock holder, member of speakers bureau, etc.). The University of Virginia School of Medicine will employ appropriate mechanisms to resolve potential conflicts of interest to maintain the standards of fair and balanced education to the reader. Questions about specific strategies can be directed to the Office of Continuing Medical Education, University of Virginia School of Medicine, Charlottesville, Virginia.

The faculty and staff of the University of Virginia Office of Continuing Medical Education have no financial affiliations to disclose.

The authors/editors listed below have identified no professional or financial affiliations for themselves or their spouse/partner:

Amar Agadi, MD; Wilma F. Bergfeld, MD, FAAD, FACP; Navid Bouzari, MD; Whitney P. Bowe, MD; Clay J. Cockerell, MD; Fran E. Cook-Bolden, MD; Dirk M. Elston, MD; Andrew G. Franks, Jr., MD, FACP; Rachel Glover (Acquisitions Editor); Marc E. Grossman, MD, FACP; Shannon Harrison, MBBS, MMED, FACD; Danielle Levine, BA; Margarita S. Lolis, MD; Kim M. Nichols, MD; Carlos Ricotti, MD; Alan R. Shalita, MD; Ravi Urbriani, MD; Andrew Wolf, MD (Test Author); and Claire Dava Wolinsky, BA.

The authors/editors listed below identified the following professional or financial affiliations for themselves or their spouse/partner:

Alice Gottlieb, MD, PhD is on the Speakers' Bureau for Amgen Inc. and Wyeth Pharmaceuticals; has consulting/advisory board agreements with Amgen, Inc., Centocor, Inc., Wyeth Pharmaceuticals, Celgene Corp., Bristol Myers Squibb Co., Beiersdorf, Inc., Abbott Labs, Roche, Sankyo, TEVA, Actelion, UCB, Novo Nordisk, Immune Control, DermiPsor, Incyte, Corgentech, PureTech, Magen Biosciences, Cytokine Pharmasciences, Inc. and Alnylam; and also has research/educational grants with Centocor, Amgen, Wyeth, Immune Control, Celgene, Incyte, Abbott, Pfizer and Novo Nordisk.

Paul T. Rose, MD, JD is a consultant for Restoration Robotics.

Neil S. Sadick, MD (Guest Editor) is on the Speakers' Bureau for Bioform, Cynosure, Solta, Sanofi-Aventis, Palomar, Cutera, Osyris, Deka, Allergan, and Suneva; is an industry funded research/investigator for Galderma and Osyris; is a consultant for Dior; is on the Advisory Committee/Board of Stiefel; and has stock/ownership in Radiancy.

Heidi Waldorf, MD is a consultant and is on the Speakers' Bureau for Medicis and Allergan; is a consultant for Procter and Gamble; and is a consultant, and is on the Speakers Bureau and Advisory Committee/Board, for Unilever/Dove.

Guy F. Webster, MD, PhD is an industry funded research/investigator and a consultant, and is on the Speakers Bureau and Advisory Committee/Board, for Galderma, Stiefel, and Medicis.

Disclosure of Discussion of Non-FDA Approved Uses for Pharmaceutical Products and/or Medical Devices
The University of Virginia School of Medicine, as an ACCME provider, requires that all faculty presenters identify and disclose any off-label uses for pharmaceutical and medical device products. The University of Virginia School of Medicine recommends that each physician fully review all the available data on new products or procedures prior to clinical use.

TO ENROLL

To enroll in the Medical Clinics of North America Continuing Medical Education program, call customer service at 1-800-654-2452 or visit us online at http://www.theclinics.com/home/cme. The CME program is available to subscribers for an additional fee of USD 205.

THE CLINICS ARE NOW AVAILABLE ONLINE!

Access your subscription at:
www.theclinics.com

Contributors

GUEST EDITOR

NEIL S. SADICK, MD
Clinical Professor of Dermatology, Weill Cornell Medical Center, New York, New York;
Sadick Dermatology, New York, New York

AUTHORS

AMAR AGADI, MD
Research Assistant, Cockerell and Associates Dermatopathology Laboratories/Dermpath
Diagnostics, Dallas, Texas

WILMA F. BERGFELD, MD, FAAD, FACP
Senior Staff, Department of Dermatology, Cleveland Clinic Foundation; Co-Director,
Department of Dermatopathology, Cleveland Clinic Foundation, Cleveland, Ohio

NAVID BOUZARI, MD
Resident, Department of Dermatology, University of Miami L. Miller School of Medicine,
Miami, Florida

WHITNEY P. BOWE, MD
Resident, Department of Dermatology, SUNY Downstate Medical Center, Brooklyn,
New York

CLAY J. COCKERELL, MD
Professor, Department of Dermatology, University of Texas Southwestern, Dallas, Texas;
Director, Cockerell and Associates Dermatopathology Laboratories/Dermpath
Diagnostics, Dallas, Texas

FRAN E. COOK-BOLDEN, MD
Director, Skin Specialty Group, New York; Clinical Assistant Professor, Department
of Dermatology, College of Physicians and Surgeons of Columbia University, New York,
New York

DIRK M. ELSTON, MD
Director, Department of Dermatology, Geisinger Medical Center, Danville, Pennsylvania

ANDREW G. FRANKS, Jr., MD, FACP
Clinical Professor, Departments of Dermatology & Medicine (Rheumatology) and Director,
Skin Lupus & Connective Tissue Disease Section, New York University School of
Medicine, New York, New York

ALICE GOTTLIEB, MD, PhD
Chair of Dermatology and Dermatologist-in-Chief, Department of Dermatology, Tufts
Medical Center, Tufts University School of Medicine, Boston, Massachusetts

MARC E. GROSSMAN, MD
Professor of Clinical Dermatology, Department of Dermatology, Columbia University, Herbert Irving Pavilion, New York, New York

SHANNON HARRISON, MBBS, MMed, FACD
Clinical Research Fellow, Department of Dermatology, Cleveland Clinic Foundation, Cleveland, Ohio

DANIELLE LEVINE, BA
Department of Dermatology, Tufts Medical Center, Tufts University School of Medicine, Boston, Massachusetts

MARGARITA S. LOLIS, MD
Department of Dermatology, SUNY Downstate Medical Center, Brooklyn, New York

KIM M. NICHOLS, MD
Skin Specialty Group, New York, New York

CARLOS RICOTTI, MD
Assistant Instructor, Department of Dermatology, University of Texas Southwestern Medical Center, Dallas, Texas, USA

PAUL T. ROSE, MD, JD
Academic Alliance in Dermatology, Tampa, Florida

ALAN R. SHALITA, MD
Chairman, Department of Dermatology, SUNY Downstate Medical Center, Brooklyn, New York

RAVI UBRIANI, MD
Assistant Professor of Clinical Dermatology, Department of Dermatology, Columbia University, Herbert Irving Pavilion, New York, New York

HEIDI WALDORF, MD
Director of Laser and Cosmetic Dermatology, Mount Sinai Medical Center; Associate Clinical Professor, Dermatology Department, Mount Sinai School of Medicine, New York, New York

GUY F. WEBSTER, MD, PhD
Clinical Professor, Department of Dermatology, Jefferson Medical College, Philadelphia, Pennsylvania; Webster Dermatology, Hockessin, Delaware

CLAIRE D. WOLINSKY, BA
Medical Student, Albany Medical College; Dermatology Fellow, Dermatology Department, Mount Sinai School of Medicine, New York, New York

Contents

IgE-mediated "allergic" disease. Experts now know that the etiology of atopic dermatitis may in fact be rooted in a loss of barrier function rather than IgE sensitivity alone. Even in more straightforward allergic skin diseases, such as urticaria and allergic contact dermatitis, evidence shows that their pathogenesis is not strictly immunologic. This article provides an overview of the major allergic skin diseases—atopic dermatitis, urticaria, and allergic contact dermatitis—focusing on recent research that has led to novel approaches in the diagnosis and treatment of these difficult conditions.

demonstrated how an organism can rapidly spread worldwide because of airline travel. Travelers are often contagious before they are aware that they have the disease, contributing to the spread. This article reviews bacterial, mycobacterial, fungal, and viral pathogens important to dermatologists.

Psoriasis is a debilitating chronic skin condition that afflicts millions of patients worldwide. Patients experiencing psoriasis report a magnitude of impaired quality of life that is often similar to that of patients who have heart failure and cancer. Many patients who have psoriasis are even themselves at risk for developing heart disease, metabolic syndrome, certain cancers, and psychiatric illness. Therefore, primary care physicians must appreciate the current psoriatic disease model and share a basic understanding of psoriasis management. This article reviews the epidemiology, clinical features, pathogenesis, comorbidities, and treatment of psoriasis, with special emphasis placed on the new class of medications, biologics, which are revolutionizing the management of the disease.

Facial papules (bumps) confront the general practitioner during every face-to-face meeting with the patient. Increased awareness and recognition of the facial papules that represent cutaneous signs of internal malignancy will allow an early, aggressive workup and treatment of any associated cancer. This article details the clinical presentation, etiology, pathologic findings, and associated malignancy for such presentations. A skin biopsy for histopathologic diagnosis is necessary to distinguish these clues to underlying malignancy from the numerous benign lesions that cause facial papules.

Venous diseases often present with characteristic cutaneous manifestations. The importance of diagnosing and treating dermatologic findings of chronic venous disease should be emphasized, because the estimated prevalence is as high as 17% in men and 40% in women. Varicose veins, which are one skin finding, are linked to chronic venous insufficiency and to the associated acute venous diseases, superficial thrombophlebitis and deep vein thrombosis. Several other cutaneous features are unique to acute or chronic diseases and should be recognized. Appropriate management of these disorders is necessary to avoid progression of disease and potential complications.

Preface

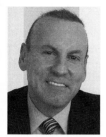

Neil S. Sadick, MD
Guest Editor

As we emerge into the twenty-first century, the diagnosis of systemic disease is reaching a new level of sophistication. In this regard, the skin is emerging as a diagnostic window of systemic disease. In addition, many patients in the arena of managed care are opting to see their primary care physician as a first line of entry into the medical system. In this setting, it is important for the primary care physician to recognize the cutaneous markers of systemic disease in order to increase the ability to treat some of the commonly encountered inflammatory dermatoses and gain increasing recognition of the diagnostic clinical signs of commonly encountered skin cancers.

In the first part of this issue of *Medical Clinics of North America*, commonly encountered inflammatory dermatoses including psoriasis acne, and rosacea are expounded upon.

The second part of the issue emphasizes diseases of the skin and nails, while the third segment discusses the cutaneous manifestations of systemic diseases and markers of internal malignancy, hypersensitivity disorders, and infectious diseases.

The final part of this issue emphasizes primary cutaneous skin cancers, venous disease sequelae, and disorders of pigmentation as commonly noted in our diverse ethnic world.

It is hoped that the present treatise will give physicians, both primary care doctors and specialists, an improved insight as to how to recognize cutaneous manifestations of internal disease and increased sophistication in the management and recognition of commonly encountered inflammatory processes and skin cancers. This knowledge will enable physicians to deliver improved patient care or provide optimal specialty-referred capabilities.

Neil S. Sadick, MD
Weill Cornell Medical Center
New York, NY
Sadick Dermatology
911 Park Avenue
Suite 1A
New York, NY 10075

E-mail address:
nssderm@sadickdermatology.com

Med Clin N Am 93 (2009) xi
doi:10.1016/j.mcna.2009.08.012
0025-7125/09/$ – see front matter © 2009 Elsevier Inc. All rights reserved.

Acne and Systemic Disease

Margarita S. Lolis, MD, Whitney P. Bowe, MD, Alan R. Shalita, MD*

KEYWORDS

- Acne • Endocrine disorders
- Acne and associated disease states
- Acne medicamentosa • Acne therapeutics

Acne vulgaris is a skin disease caused by changes in pilosebaceous units. It is common in adolescence and may proceed into adulthood, affecting roughly 33% of people between the ages of 15 and 44 years.[1] Its cutaneous manifestations are well known to clinicians and have been amply described. The endocrine causes and associated disease states are less commonly described and less well known to general clinicians and are emphasized in this article. Nonendocrine diseases of which acne is a feature are also discussed, along with pharmaceutical causes of acne and acneiform drug eruptions.

HORMONES AND ACNE

Sebaceous gland activity and sebum production play a central role in the development of acne. The sebaceous gland is hormonally regulated. Several hormones have been linked to acne and may regulate sebaceous secretion. They include androgens, estrogens, growth hormone, insulin, insulin growth factor 1 (IGF-1), corticotropin-releasing hormone (CRF), adrenocorticotropic hormone (ACTH), melanocortins, and glucocorticoids.

Androgens

Androgens are one of the most important classes of hormones implicated in the pathophysiology of acne. Most circulating androgens are produced by the adrenal glands and gonads, are involved in regulating many systemic processes, and play a major role in the skin. In addition to being synthesized by endocrine organs, these hormones are also produced by the skin, where all of the necessary enzymes required for the conversion from cholesterol to steroids are located.[2] Their effects are exerted mainly on the sebaceous gland, where androgen receptors have been localized to the basal

No financial disclosures.
Department of Dermatology, SUNY Downstate Medical Center, 450 Clarkson Avenue, Brooklyn, NY 11203, USA
* Corresponding author.
E-mail address: alan.shalita@downstate.edu (A.R. Shalita).

Med Clin N Am 93 (2009) 1161–1181
doi:10.1016/j.mcna.2009.08.008
0025-7125/09/$ – see front matter © 2009 Elsevier Inc. All rights reserved.

layer of the sebaceous gland and the outer root sheath of the hair follicle.[3–5] Androgens have been shown to trigger sebaceous gland growth and development and to stimulate sebum production.[6–9]

Clinical evidence supports the link between androgen and acne formation. Sebum production increases markedly during the prepubertal period, a time when serum levels of dihydroepiandrosterone sulfate (DHEAS), a precursor to testosterone, are also elevated. Individuals who are insensitive to androgen do not produce sebum and do not develop acne, and high androgen states are associated with acne formation.[2] In some studies, acne patients have higher circulating levels of free testosterone,[7] DHEAS,[2] 5α-reductase,[2,6] and androgen receptors in the sebaceous gland[6] compared with patients without acne. It is commonly believed, however, that hypersensitivity of the sebaceous glands to androgens is the underlying cause of acne.[2,7]

The exact mechanism by which androgens promote sebaceous gland activity and hypertrophy is unclear but scientific evidence supports this association.[2,8–12] Testosterone and dihydrotestosterone (DHT) bind nuclear androgen receptors, which then interact with deoxyribonucleic acid (DNA) in the nucleus of sebaceous cells and ultimately regulate genes involved in cell proliferation and lipogenesis.[8–10] Although these exact target genes are not known, they may include genes that encode growth factors and lipogenic enzymes.[2] Peroxisome proliferator-activated receptor (PPAR) ligands may also be implicated in regulation of lipid metabolic genes.[2,11,12]

Estrogens

The major active estrogen, estradiol, is synthesized from testosterone by the aromatase enzyme, which is active in adipose tissue and in the skin.[2] In contrast to testosterone, estradiol decreases sebum production in supraphysiological doses.[13] The dose of ethinyl estradiol commonly found in current oral contraceptive pills (OCPs) is not sufficient to demonstrate a reduction in sebum secretion.[13] However, there are no recent studies to confirm this observation. As some acne patients respond well to the lower-dose OCPs, various mechanisms have been proposed to explain this effect. They include: (1) inhibition of gonadal testosterone production through negative feedback suppression of gonadotropins[2,10]; (2) increased production of sex hormone binding globulin (SHBG) by the liver, thereby decreasing free serum testosterone[2,9,11]; (3) direct opposition of androgen within the sebaceous gland[2,8,9]; and (4) gene regulation of sebaceous gland growth and lipid production.[2,9,14]

Growth Hormone

Growth hormone (GH) is secreted by the pituitary gland and stimulates production of IGFs in the liver and peripheral tissues.[2] GH is thought to play a role in acne development directly and indirectly through IGF-1 stimulation.

Clinical observations suggest that GH may influence acne formation.[2,15] In a pattern similar to androgen, the natural course of acne from its onset in puberty to its peak in mid-adolescence and subsequent decline corresponds to levels of GH. Furthermore, conditions of GH excess, such as acromegaly, are associated with acne development and sebum overproduction.[2,15]

The role of GH in acne development may be mediated through its effect on the sebaceous gland. The GH receptor is found in hair follicles and the acini of sebaceous glands.[15] Animal studies have shown that GH can stimulate growth of sebocyte-containing preputial glands[16] and that androgen-induced sebum production may be mediated through GH.[17] In vitro studies have shown that GH directly stimulates sebocyte differentiation and augments the effects of DHT on sebaceous gland differentiation.[13] Furthermore, atrophic preputial glands, composed mostly of sebocytes, cannot be restored to normal size with testosterone alone, but do show growth when supplemented with GH.[18] The preputial gland, however, is not precisely comparable to human sebaceous glands.

IGF-1

GH stimulates IGF-1 production. Women with acne have significantly higher levels of IGF-1 compared with women without acne.[2,15,18] Like GH, the incidence of acne strongly correlates to levels of IGF-1.[2,15,18] A positive correlation between serum IGF-1 levels and facial sebum levels has been reported.[19]

IGF plays a role in acne through its effects on androgens, sebaceous gland growth, and lipogenesis. These roles are supported by the following scientific evidence:

1. IGF-1 has the ability to stimulate adrenal androgen synthesis and inhibit the production of hepatic SHBG, which leads to a subsequent increase in free androgen.[20]
2. IGF-1 induces sebocyte proliferation by stimulating DNA synthesis.[18] IGF-1 receptors are expressed in hair follicles and peripheral cells of the sebaceous gland.[15] Because these receptors are located where basal highly mitotic cells of the gland reside, there is a possibility that IGF-1 may directly stimulate the sebaceous epithelium by acting as a trophic factor.[15]
3. IGF-1 stimulates sebaceous gland lipogenesis by increasing expression of the transcriptions factor sterol response element binding protein-1, which regulates key genes involved in lipid biosynthesis.[20]

Insulin

Insulin is structurally related to IGF-1 and can bind to the IGF-1 receptor.[15] Although it most likely acts as a mixed IGF-1 agonist/antagonist, its direct effects on sebocytes are distinct from IGF-1. In very high doses, insulin up-regulates GH receptor expression on sebocytes, thereby potentiating GH-induced differentiation.[15] In addition, insulin may act as a key regulator of lipid biosynthetic enzymes[18] by stimulating ovarian and adrenal androgen production and inhibiting hepatic SHBG production. Insulin decreases IGF binding protein, which maximizes free IGF-1 concentrations to act on target tissues[20] and increases testosterone bioavailability and DHEAS concentrations.[21–24] The role of diet in acne is controversial, but recent studies support an association. It has been proposed that high foods with a high glycemic load (HGL) elevate plasma insulin concentrations, which regulates levels of androgen, IGF-1 and IGF binding protein, promotes unregulated tissue growth, and enhances androgen synthesis.[25] A randomized controlled trial comparing a diet with a low glycemic load (LGL) to a conventional HGL diet demonstrated greater improvement of acne and insulin sensitivity in patients who followed an LGL diet compared with a conventional HGL diet.[20] Another study demonstrated that LGL decreases total lesion counts, decreases follicular sebum outflow, and changes the composition of skin surface triglycerides,[23] further supporting a causal link between insulin and acne.

Corticotropin-releasing Hormone

Corticotropin-releasing hormone (CRH) is secreted by the hypothalamus and binds to receptors of the anterior pituitary, which in turn, synthesizes propiomelanocortin (POMC). POMC is degraded into ACTH and melanocyte-stimulating hormone (MSH), and ultimately regulates cortisol production.[14]

In the skin, a complete CRH, CRH binding protein (CRHBP) and CRH receptor system has been elucidated by in vivo and in vitro studies.[14,26] CRH is released by dermal nerves and sebocytes in response to proinflammatory cytokines[10] and stimulates its receptors in paracrine and autocrine fashions. The main cutaneous target of CRH is the sebaceous gland. CRH has numerous functions: it inhibits sebaceous proliferation, promotes sebaceous differentiation, and induces sebaceous gland lipogenesis by enhancing androgen bioavailability.[27] It also interacts with testosterone and GH through a complex regulatory system and stimulates conversion of DHEA to testosterone. CRH expression is up-regulated in acne-involved sebaceous glands in vivo compared with noninvolved sebaceous glands of acne patients and sebaceous glands of healthy individuals.[28] Clinical and experiment evidence implicates the involvement of CRH in the development of acne.[29]

Melanocortins

POMC is produced by the anterior pituitary in response to CRH from the hypothalamus. POMC is broken down into the melanocortins ACTH and MSH. Human sebocytes express the melanocortin receptors MC-1R and MC-5R, through which ACTH and MSH regulate various effects on the sebaceous gland.[22,26,30] MC-1R may be involved in immunoregulation, as studies have shown that MSH suppresses secretion of interleukin 8, a central proinflammatory mediator in acne vulgaris.[30] Expression of MC-1R is also increased in sebaceous glands of lesional skin of patients with acne.[31] MC-5R is thought to be involved in sebocyte differentiation and lipogenesis.[26] Mice that lack the MC-5R exhibit decreased sebum production.[2]

Glucocorticoids

Cortisol, the main glucocorticoid in humans, is a stress hormone under the direct regulation of ACTH. It is well known that use of topical or systemic glucocorticoids promotes an acneiform eruption.[32] This observation suggests a role of cortisol in sebaceous functioning. In vitro studies demonstrate that hydrocortisone stimulates sebocyte proliferation in a dose-dependent manner, and that cortisol is essential for sebocyte differentiation, necessary for GH and IGF-1 induced sebocyte differentiation and IGF-1 mediated proliferation. These results suggest that steroid-induced acne may be due to its promotion of sebocyte proliferation and differentiation.[15] Long-term use of oral glucocorticoids is also known to exacerbate inflammatory lesions in acne vulgaris. This effect may be mediated through steroid-induced activation of toll-like receptor 2 (TLR2), a proinflammatory mediator.[32]

ENDOCRINE DISORDERS ASSOCIATED WITH ACNE

Many hormones are implicated in acne formation through their regulation of sebaceous gland growth, development, and activity. Diseases with overproduction of any of these hormones are therefore associated with acne. Polycystic ovarian syndrome, Cushing syndrome, congenital adrenal hyperplasia, androgen-secreting tumors, and acromegaly are examples of endocrine causes of acne.

Polycystic Ovarian Syndrome

Polycystic ovary syndrome (PCOS) is the most common hormonal disorder in young women. Its diagnosis relies upon the presence of two out of the three following criteria: (1) oligomennorrhea or amenorrhea; (2) hyperandrogenism (clinical evidence of androgen excess) or hyperandrogenemia (biochemical evidence of androgen excess); or (3) polycystic ovaries as demonstrated by ultrasound.[33] The main abnormality in PCOS is increased ovarian production of androgens, which is mostly likely caused by abnormal regulation of 17α-hydroxylase, the rate-limiting enzyme in androgen biosynthesis.[34] The excess ovarian androgens act locally to cause ovarian dysfunction and peripherally to cause acne and other signs of hyperandrogenism such as hirsutism and androgenic alopecia.[34] In peripheral adipose tissue, excess androgens are converted to estrogen in an acyclic manner, which causes an increase in pituitary secretion of luteinizing hormone (LH). Peripheral insulin resistance is also evident in women with PCOS, and the resulting hyperinsulinemia contributes to increased ovarian hypersecretion of androgens and direct stimulation of pituitary LH production.[34]

Approximately 23% to 35% of women with PCOS have acne and the majority of women with severe acne have PCOS, with reported rates as high as 83%.[33] These women also present with infertility or menstrual irregularities caused by anovulatory cycles, obesity, diabetes, and hirsutism.[2] PCOS should be suspected in patients with late-onset acne, persistent acne, and acne resistant to conventional therapies. Acne formation is likely related to abnormally elevated androgen and insulin levels.

As PCOS is mainly a diagnosis of exclusion, other conditions that cause irregular menses or androgen excess must first be excluded. These conditions may include late-onset congenital adrenal hyperplasia, Cushing syndrome, adrenal or ovarian androgen-secreting tumors, or drugs.[33]

PCOS may be subtle and variable in presentation, necessitating an individualized approach for evaluation. Evaluation should commence with a comprehensive history of the patient's menstrual cycle, problems with infertility or miscarriage, and signs of hyperandrogenism. Use of oral contraception may mask menstrual irregularities and hyperandrogenism and should always be considered and questioned.[2,33] A family history of PCOS, diabetes mellitus, and hyperandrogenism should be elicited.

Physical examination is focused on signs and symptoms of androgen excess, including hirsutism, acne, seborrhea, acanthosis nigricans, clitoromegaly, deepening of the voice, increased muscle mass, and decreased breast size.[33] Screening laboratory tests to evaluate for hyperandrogenism are recommended and include serum DHEAS, total testosterone, free testosterone, and luteinizing hormone/follicle stimulating hormone (LH/FSH ratio).[33] For patients who are on OCPs, discontinuation for 4 to 6 weeks before endocrine evaluation is optimal.[2] Free testosterone is the most sensitive test for hyperandrogenemia and is a marker for ovarian androgens.[33] One-third of patients with PCOS have elevated levels of total and free testosterone (**Table 1**). DHEAS is elevated in 20% of white PCOS patients and sometimes may be the only abnormal laboratory finding.[33] These serum levels do not exceed 700 µg/dL, but when they do, an androgen-secreting tumor should be considered. Elevated levels of LH are found in 40% to 90% of women with PCOS and is almost pathognomic for this disease.[33] FSH levels are within normal range but the LH/FSH ratio is greater than 3 in up to 95% of patients.[33] Since LH and FSH are variable during different phases of the menstrual cycle, they have a low sensitivity for diagnosing PCOS.[33] These samples are best drawn at a time in the menstrual cycle that does not correspond to the time of ovulation (as close to menses as possible).

Fasting glucose and insulin levels, markers of impaired glucose tolerance, which are elevated in 30% to 45% of PCOS patients, are not diagnostic but recommended in these patients because of the association of diabetes mellitus type 2 and PCOS.[33]

Treatment of acne in patients with PCOS involves reducing androgen levels or blocking the effects of androgens on the sebaceous gland. The first-line therapy, therefore, is treatment with OCPs. The estrogen in OCPs reduces LH and ovarian androgen production, increases liver synthesis of SHBG, thereby lowering levels of free testosterone and DHEAS, and directly reduces sebum production. Choice of progestin is important when prescribing an OCP, as some of them have

Table 1
Endocrine abnormalities in acne-associated endocrine disorders

	DHEAS (Plasma ng/mL)	Total Testosterone (Plasma ng/dl)	17-OH Progesterone (Plasma ng/mL)	Cortisol (Urine μg/24 h)[a]	LH/FSH
Normal range	500–2500	20–90	0.2–1	20–90	2
PCOS	Normal/ slightly increased	100–200	Normal	Normal	2–3
CAH	4000–8000	100–200	>3	Normal	Normal
Adrenal tumor	>8000	>200	Normal/ increased	Normal/>90	Normal
Cushing syndrome	Normal	100–200	Normal/ increased	>90	Normal
Androgen- secreting tumor	>700	>200	Normal	Normal	Normal

[a] Radioimmunoassay (RIA).
Data from Refs.[98–101]

antiandrogenic effects. It is commonly believed that certain progesterones may have proandrogenic effects, but this concept is currently being questioned (A.R. Shalita and J.J. Leyden, personal communication, December 2008). Some oral contraceptives have been approved by the US Food and Drug Administration (FDA) for the treatment of acne vulgaris, and clinical data are available to support the use of several other brands (see **Box 1**).

Other antiandrogenic treatments include spironolactone and flutamide. Sprinolactone is a potassium-sparing diuretic that decreases ovarian and adrenal androgen production and blocks androgen actions at the receptor level. It is synergistic when combined with OCPs. Flutamide selectively blocks nuclear androgen receptors. Although it is used mostly to treat hirsutism, it has been shown to be superior to

Box 1
Oral contraceptives and the treatment of acne vulgaris

FDA-approved brands for the treatment of acne vulgaris

Estrostrep

Ortho Tri-Cyclen

Yaz

Clinical data are available to support the use of the following brands:

Alesse

Diane-35[a]

Yasmin.

[a] Not available in the United States.

spironolactone in the management of acne.[35] Flutamide is not commonly used to treat acne because of the risk for hepatotoxicity.

Lifestyle modifications are paramount for the management of insulin resistance in PCOS patients. An LGL diet has been shown to increase insulin sensitivity[20,23–25] and SHBG levels,[36] decrease testosterone levels,[36] and improve acne,[20,23–25] but has yet to be specifically studied among patients with PCOS. Metformin has been shown to reduce insulin and testosterone levels and improve acne in PCOS patients with or without insulin resistance.[37] In the authors' opinion, metformin alone is ineffective, but can be helpful when used in combination with OCPs.

Cushing Syndrome

Cushing syndrome results from an excess of glucocorticoid secretion. Causes of Cushing syndrome may be ACTH dependent or independent and include pituitary hypersecretion of ACTH, ectopic secretion of ACTH by nonpituitary tumors, CRH secreting tumors, bilateral adrenal hyperplasia, and adrenocortical adenoma or carcinomas that autonomously secrete cortisol.[38]

Many skin changes occur with Cushing syndrome including acne. These acne lesions are typically monomorphic, perifollicular papules produced by hyperkeratosis of follicular openings usually on the face, chest, and back. Mild pustule formation can be seen but deep cystic lesions and comedo formation characteristic of adolescent acne is uncommon. The pathophysiology of acne formation in the context of Cushing syndrome may be related to abnormalities in levels of CRH, ACTH, and cortisol. These hormones stimulate sebaceous growth and development, promote lipogenesis and sebum production, and increase levels of testosterone.[2,14,38]

Congenital Adrenal Hyperplasia

Congenital adrenal hyperplasia (CAH) results from impaired steroid synthesis by the adrenal cortex because of genetic enzyme deficiencies.[39] The most common enzyme deficiency is 21-hydroxylase deficiency, followed by 11-hydroxylase deficiency. Deficiencies in these enzymes result in the shunting of steroids from the cortisol biosynthetic pathway to the androgen biosynthetic pathway. Adequate levels of cortisol exist but excessive amounts of adrenal androgens are produced.

21-Hydroxylase deficiency is classified as classic or nonclassic.[40] In the classic form, there is complete deficiency of the enzyme so that the hyperandrogenism is more severe and manifests as ambiguous genitalia in females. These patients have an early and severe onset of acne, especially cystic acne, and other signs of virilization.[39] In the milder nonclassic form, in which there is only a partial defect of the enzyme, symptoms of hyperandrogenism are not apparent at birth and ambiguous genitalia in females are not present.[33,39,40]

Acne may be the only presenting symptom of CAH in the nonclassic form.[1,41,42] Of these patients, 33% present with acne.[40] In men with severe acne, CAH may be underestimated as other symptoms are usually masked. Although some studies recommend screening for the presence of nonclassic CAH in young men presenting with acne alone,[43,44] this is not widely practiced by clinicians.

Children or adolescents with early and severe onset of acne, pubic hair, rapid growth, amenorrhea, or any signs of androgen excess, should be evaluated for CAH. Serum levels of DHEAS can be used to screen for adrenal androgen excess,[2] with values typically ranging from 4000 to 8000 ng/mL. A high concentration of 17-hydroxyprogesterone (>242 nmol/L, >3 ng/mL) is diagnostic for classic CAH.[2] In nonclassic CAH, a corticotropin stimulation test with measurement of 17-hydroxyprogesterone at 60 minutes is the gold standard.[40] A stimulated 17-hydroxyprogesterone concentration higher than 45 nmol/L is diagnostic.[40] Treatment is targeted to correcting the underlying deficiency. Glucocorticoid replacement corrects the deficiency and hyperandrogenic symptoms by suppressing the inappropriately activated hypothalamic-pituitary-adrenal axis. Low-dose prednisone (2.5–5 mg at bedtime, or dexamethasone 0.25–0.5 mg daily) are typically used. In terms of acne therapy, female patients with CAH and acne may also benefit from antiandrogen treatments such as oral contraceptives, spironolactone, or flutamide.[45] A study of 20 females with nonclassic CAH demonstrated reversal of their acne after 3 months of therapy with dexamethasone (0.25 mg/d).[38,45,46]

Androgen-secreting Tumors

Androgen-secreting tumors may be adrenal, ovarian, or testicular in origin and are exceedingly rare, accounting for only 0.2% of the causes of androgen excess ([47,48]; **Table 2**). An abrupt onset of acne vulgaris with comedone formation is suspicious of an androgen-secreting tumor.[38] However, some androgen-secreting tumors may produce only moderate levels of androgens and therefore, have a more indolent presentation.[47]

Adrenocortical carcinomas typically present with a mixed picture of Cushing syndrome with virilization.[42] Even rarer are adrenal tumors that solely produce androgen and no cortisol, and present purely with virilization.[42] Androgen-secreting tumors of the ovary present similarly, again with symptoms of hyperandrogenism in females, including hirsutism, virilization, and menstrual abnormalities. Distinction between the two types of androgen-secreting tumors is based on laboratory findings and radiologic techniques.[42]

Serum levels of DHEAS, total testosterone, free testosterone, LH, and FSH should be ordered to screen for all causes of hyperandrogenism. DHEAS is used to screen for an adrenal source of excess androgens, and an elevated serum level of total testosterone is suspicious for an ovarian or testicular source. A serum level of DHEAS

Table 2		
Androgen-secreting tumors of the gonads and the adrenals		
Ovarian	**Testicular**[a]	**Adrenal**
Sex cord-stromal tumors:	Stromal tumors:	Adrenal adenomas
Sertoli-Leydig cell	Leydig cell tumor	Adrenal carcinomas
tumors	Sertoli cell tumor	
Granulosa-theca cell	Sertoli-Leydig cell	
tumors	tumors	
Lipoid or lipid cell tumors:	Germ cell tumors:	
Hilar cell type	Seminomas	
	Yolk sac tumors	
	Teratomas	
	Choriocarcinomas	
Gonadoblastomas	Gonadoblastomas:	
	Germ cell and stroma cell	

[a] Testicular tumors can cause enhanced production of testosterone or estradiol, presenting as virilization or feminization.

Data from Carr BR. Disorders of the ovaries and female reproductive tract. In: Wilson JD, Foster DW, Kronenberg HM, et al, editors. Williams textbook of endocrinology. 9th edition. Philadelphia: WB Saunders Company; 1998. p. 798; Griffin JE, Wilson JD. Disorders of the testes and the male reproductive tract. In: Wilson JD, Foster DW, Kronenberg HM, et al, editors. Williams textbook of endocrinology. 9th edition. Philadelphia: WB Saunders Company; 1998. p. 852.

greater than 8000 ng/mL may be indicative of an adrenal tumor and should be further evaluated. An ovarian or testicular tumor is associated with serum levels of total testosterone exceeding 200 ng/dL.[49]

Acromegaly

Acromegaly, a condition of GH excess, is associated with the development of acne.[2] Since the progression of this disorder can be slow, reliance on clinical signs is paramount for early diagnosis. Reports of acne vulgaris as the only presenting symptom of acromegaly have been published,[50] and sebum production has been shown to be increased in patients with acromegaly.[51] These effects may be due to excess levels of GH and IGF-1, which stimulate sebaceous gland growth and differentiation, and androgen-induced sebaceous lipogenesis.[15,18,51]

ASSOCIATED DISEASE STATES

Acne is a feature of several nonendocrine diseases described in the following sections. The clinical appearance of acne may help guide or suggest the diagnosis in several of these disorders, as other disease manifestations may be subtle.

Apert Syndrome

Apert syndrome, also known as acrocephalosyndactyly type I is a rare autosomal dominant congenital disorder caused by a mutation in the gene encoding the fibroblast growth factor receptor.[52] This receptor is responsible for the development of the embryonic skeleton, epithelial structures, and connective tissue.[53] Therefore, mutations in this gene cause premature obliteration of the craniofacial sutures and syndactyly of the hands and feet.[54]

Clinically, these patients present with different craniofacial deformities, hypertelorism, dental abnormalities, and proptosis of the eyes.[53] Pilosebaceous abnormalities in these patients have also been described. Early appearance of widespread and severe acne resistant to conventional therapies is a common clinical feature of this disorder.[54]

The dermatologic hallmark of Apert syndrome is severe inflammatory and comedonal acne involving the face, chest, back, and unusual sites such as the forearms, buttocks, and thighs.[55] Forearm acne has been observed in 70% of patients with Apert syndrome; it usually develops at puberty between the ages of 9 and 12 years.[56] Immunohistochemical staining of sebocyte androgen receptors showed no difference in number of cells with androgen receptor expression between patients with Apert syndrome and normal control patients.[57] Therefore, the underlying abnormality may be associated with increased sensitivity to normal circulating levels of androgens of certain tissues and organs.[56,57] This hyperresponse to androgens, which may be mediated by ketarinocyte growth factor receptors, may also explain premature epiphyseal fusion.[54,57,58]

Management of acne in patients with Apert syndrome is challenging, as these patients are unresponsive to conventional therapy.[52] Isotretinoin has been reported to be successful in treating acne in these patients. Although some dermatologists believe that aggressive treatment with higher dosages of isotretinoin (>1 mg/kg/d) is more beneficial, treatment with 1 mg/kg/d has been shown to be adequate but it usually requires a more protracted course.[52,55]

Synovitis Acne Pustulosis Hyperostosis Osteitis Syndrome

Synovitis acne pustulosis hyperostosis osteitis (SAPHO) syndrome is characterized clinically by any combination of synovitis, acne, pustulosis, hyperostosis, and osteitis.[59] The cause of this rare disease is unknown and it is observed primarily in children, young adults, or middle-aged individuals.[59] Chronic multifocal recurrent osteomyelitis is a common feature of this disease and mostly affects the sternum, pelvis, lower jaw, and clavicles. The osteomyelitis is usually sterile or may show presence of *Propionibacterium acnes*.[59]

Skin lesions in SAPHO syndrome are characterized by severe acne fulminans or acne conglobata, palmoplantar pustulosis, or pustular psoriasis.[59] Skin biopsy reveals neutrophilic pseudoabscesses.[60] Only 60% of patients are reported to have skin involvement and may present 2 to 20 years after bone involvement.[59] On rare occasions, skin manifestations may be very subtle.

The SAPHO syndrome should be suspected in patients with inflammatory skin diseases with any bone or musculoskeletal symptoms and who satisfy one of the following clinical diagnostic criteria: (1) oseoarticular manifestations of acne conglobata, acne fulminans, or hidradenitis suppurativa; (2) osteoarticular manifestations of palmoplantar pustulosis; (3) axial or appendicular hyperostosis with or without dermatosis; or (4) chronic recurrent multifocal osteomyelitis involving the axial or appendicular skeleton with or without a dermatosis.[52] To manage musculoskeletal symptoms, steroidal and nonsteroidal antiinflammatory drugs are the mainstay of therapy. For acne and palmoplantar pustulosis, retinoids are frequently used. For severe acne, isotretinoin has been effective. Infliximab has also been used with success.[61]

Behçet Syndrome

Recurrent oral and genital ulcerations and uveitis are the originally described clinical hallmarks of Behçet syndrome. Multisystem involvement in this syndrome has subsequently been described to include the skin, articular, gastrointestinal, and central nervous system. The basic pathologic process in Behçet syndrome is vasculitis involving the arterial and venous system. The etiology of this syndrome is unknown but it is associated with the human lymphocyte antigen-B51 (HLA-B51) allele, especially among Asian patients.[62]

The acne lesions characteristic of Behçet syndrome are usually observed in combination with arthritis. The individual lesions are indistinguishable from acne vulgaris clinically and histologically. The preferred sites differ, with the arms and legs being more commonly involved; the face, chest, neck, back, and hairline of patients may also be involved.[62] The acne lesions are not sterile and their microbiology is similar to acne vulgaris.[63] The presence of the acne lesions may be associated with the pathogenesis of the disease, as a pustule or papule typically forms 24 to 48 hours after a pathergy test. Other skin manifestations include nodular lesions, either erythema nodosum or superficial thrombophlebitis, which are see in about 50% of patients with Behçet syndrome.[62]

Treatment is challenging, and multiple therapies may be used to induce remissions. Colchicine, dapsone, and oral prednisone are frequently used, and treatment with tumor necrosis factor inhibitors, such as infliximab, has also been used successfully.[64] In general, many patients with Behçet syndrome achieve complete remission.

PAPA Syndrome

PAPA syndrome is an autoinflammatory disorder characterized by pyogenic arthritis, pyoderma gangrenosum, and acne. It is inherited in an autosomal dominant fashion and is caused by a mutation in the CD2 binding protein 1 (CD2BP1), which has been identified on chromosome 15.[65,66] The mechanism of action of the mutated gene is still under investigation. PAPA syndrome manifests clinically during childhood with recurrent and destructive arthritis.[66] Pyoderma gangeronsum does not always present in affected individuals.

However, acne does affect most individuals with PAPA syndrome and is usually severe nodulocystic acne. It begins in adolescence and proceeds into adulthood.[65] Management of this disorder is challenging. Treatment of acne usually requires isotretinoin.[65,66]

ACNE MEDICAMENTOSA

By definition, acne medicamentosa is acne caused or aggravated by medications. Since acne is a disorder of the pilosebaceous unit that is hormonally regulated, exogenous hormones such as danazol and testosterone can trigger acne. Other systemic drugs can cause acne or acneiform eruptions including lithium, isoniazid, phenytoin, vitamins B_2, B_6, and B_{12}, halogens, and EGFR inhibitors. Unlike acne vulgaris, drug-induced acne is characterized by a monomorphic eruption of papules and pustules, and classically involves the trunk rather than the face. Open and closed comedones are typically absent. A sudden onset of acne vulgaris or an acneiform eruption in association with the following medications is suspicious for acne medicamentosa (**Box 2**).

Glucocorticoids

Glucocorticoid therapy is a well-known trigger of acne, commonly referred to as steroid acne. It differs from acne vulgaris in its distribution and in the types of lesions observed. It is characterized by small pustules and papules that are all at the same stage of development.[49] The lesions usually appear on the trunk, shoulders, and upper arms and seldomly involve the face unless topical steroids are directly applied to the face. In this case, perioral acne or steroid rosacea may result, manifesting as inflamed papules and pustules on an erythematous background. A follicular eruption may appear as early as 2 weeks after initiation of systemic or topical steroids.[49] On histology, steroid acne is characterized by a focal folliculitis with a neutrophilic infiltrate in and around the hair follicle.[49] Discontinuation of the steroid is the primary treatment, but conventional acne treatments including retinoid and antibiotics are also beneficial.

Box 2
Drugs capable of inducing acne and acneiform eruptions
Drug
Danazol
Testosterone
Progestins
Glucocorticoids
Lithium
Isoniazid
Phenytoin
Vitamins B_2, B_6, and B_{12}
Halogens
EGFR inhibitors

Progestins

Eight forms of synthetic progestins are used in OCPs with varying amount of androgenic activity. These progestins are thought to cross-react with androgen receptors, and could potentially aggravate acne. The third-generation progestins, including norgestimate, desogestrel, and gestodene, are more selective for the progesterone receptor. Regardless of their potential to cross-react with androgen receptors, almost all oral contraceptives have proven beneficial in the treatment of acne. Thus, the progestin effects are likely offset by the estrogen effects of the combination pills. Several combination OCPs are currently approved by the FDA for the treatment of acne (see **Box 1**). Drospirenone, a progestin derived from spironolactone, has antiandrogenic (treats acne) and antimineralocorticoid (treats bloating/acts as a diuretic) activity. Drospirenone is found is Yaz and Yasmin. The long-acting subdermal implant, Norplant (Bayer Schering Pharma AG, Berlin, Germany), consists of norgestrel, and acne is a common complaint among female users. Flaring of acne in females using Norplant is variable and unpredictable.[67]

Lithium

Lithium aggravates cutaneous conditions histologically characterized by neutrophilic infiltration.[68] Acne vulgaris and acneiform eruptions are two such conditions. Lithium may stimulate neutrophils, which play a central role in the inflammatory acne.[69] Acne lesions may involve typical sites of acne vulgaris but may also be present on the legs and arms. Classically, cysts and comedones are not present. Onset may occur with initial use or after increasing the dose of the drug or may present as a flare in existing disease.[70]

Controlled studies of the adverse side effects of lithium demonstrate that acne may affect 33% to 45% of patients treated with lithium,[68,71] with a stronger predisposition for men. This may be related to increased levels of testosterone in men.[68] Management of acne in these patients involves treatment with topical or oral antibiotics. Treatment is usually effective[68–71] but occasionally patients may be less responsive, particularly if they remain on high doses of lithium.[70] Use of topical tretinoin has been successful. Improvement of lesions is variable and they may subside with or without reduction in dosage or cessation of lithium.[70]

Isoniazid

Isoniazid is known to cause an acneiform eruption consisting of inflammatory pustules with open and closed comedones. The onset is abrupt and there is greater predominance of comedones than inflammatory lesions. Patients who are slow acetylators are more commonly affected.[69]

Phenytoin

The antiepilectic drug phenytoin causes increased levels of testosterone, resulting in hyperandrogenism.[72] Phenytoin is thought to cause or aggravate acne through its androgenic effect, which ultimately stimulates the pilosebaceous unit.[72–74] In one study, 80.3% of patients on phenytoin developed acne compared with 30.2% in nonepilectic females.[73,74]

Vitamins B_2, B_6, and B_{12}

Vitamins B_2 (riboflavin), B_6 (pyridoxine), and B_{12} (cyanocobalamin) may trigger or exacerbate acne or aceniform eruptions.[75] The lesions appear acutely after initial treatment[76] and consist of small papules or pustules on the face, back, chest, and upper arms.[77] All age groups are affected, with a predisposition for females. The eruption fades rapidly upon discontinuation of the vitamin.[77] The etiologic and pathogenic mechanism is not known.[76] Several cases of an eruption resembling acne rosacea have been reported after ingestion of high-dose vitamin B supplement. The eruption did not respond to standard rosacea treatment but disappeared quickly after discontinuation of the supplement.[78]

Halogens

Exposure to compounds that contain halogens may cause acne. Such industrial compounds include chlorinated hydrocarbons, coal tar derivatives, and insoluble cutting oils. Other halogens are iodides and bromides, which are found in thyroid and asthma medications.[49,69]

Chloracne describes acne that results from chlorinated hydrocarbons. It is characteristically composed of numerous large comedones, cysts, nodules, papules and pustules involving the face, neck, axilla, penis, and scrotum or any area that comes into contact. Chlorinated hydrocarbons are found in fungicides, insecticides, and wood preservatives. The disease is often chronic as chemicals are deposited in adipose tissue. Lesions take up to 2 years to clear once exposure to the chemical has been terminated and adipose tissue stores have been cleared.[49]

Iododerma refers to skin lesions caused by exposure to substances with iodine. Tender pustules that coalesce into crusting plaques and nodules are the hallmark of iododerma. The face, along with regions high in sebaceous activity, is primarily affected. Antibiotics and removal of the offending agent are beneficial. The underlying pathologic mechanism is unknown; however, eosinophilia has been associated with iododerma. Intradermal skin testing with iodides is negative. Iodide-induced destabilization of mast cells leading to eosinophilia may be implicated in the pathogenesis.[69]

EGRF Inhibitors

EGFR inhibitors are a class of antineoplastic drugs that includes gefitnib, cetuximab, erlotinib, and trastuzumab. EGFR inhibitors are commonly used in the treatment of carcinomas of the lung, breast, and colon. A perifollicular, papulopustular eruption on the face and upper torso is frequently associated with use of these drugs and is used to assess response to the drug clinically.[49] Such an acneiform eruption portends a good response to the drug, and a favorable prognosis for the patient.[79] Comedones are not present.[80] It occurs as quickly as 7 days after initiation of treatment[80] and affects up to 86% of patients.[49] The perifolliculitis is noninfectious, and although the etiology is not completely understood, it is thought to result directly from EGFR blockade of the hair follicle.[81] Rapid response to conventional acne treatments such as benzoyl peroxide, retinoids, and topical or oral antibiotics has been reported.[80,81]

GENERAL BASIC THERAPEUTIC INTERVENTIONS

The principal goal of acne therapy is the reduction or elimination of all acne lesions and their precursors, microcomedones. Four general categories of medications have proven efficacious for the treatment of acne: (1) topical therapy; (2) systemic antibiotics; (3) hormonal agents; and (4) isotretinoin. Treatment with these agents is dependent on severity of acne disease.

Topical Therapy

Topical therapy is considered first-line therapy for acne[82] and is indicated in patients with noninflammatory comedones or mild-to-moderate inflammatory acne.[83] Comedolytic agents primarily target comedones and antibacterials and antibiotics target inflammatory lesions. Recent evidence suggests that the effects of antibacterials on TLR2s may explain the reduction in comedones seen in most clinical trials with antibacterials.[84] Topical retinoids (tretinoin, adapalene, and tazarotene), normalize the follicular differentiation, which leads to the follicular obstruction causing microcomedones, the precursor of other acne lesions.[82] This normalization reverses abnormal keratinization,[82] which affects microcomedones, open and closed comedones, and inflammatory lesions. Topical retinoids may also improve postinflammatory hyperpigmentation but may be locally irritating.[83]

Benzoyl peroxide (BP) is a bactericidal agent with the ability to prevent or eliminate skin colonization with *P acnes*.[83] It improves noninflammatory and inflammatory lesions and is used in combination with oral or topical antibiotics to reduce bacterial resistance.[82] Topical antibiotics are used for inflammatory lesions and most frequently include clindamyin and erythromycin.[82] Decreased microbial sensitivity to these agents is a limitation to their use as monotherapy. Combination with BP is beneficial not only because it reduces rates of *P acnes* resistance but also because it exerts a synergistic antimicrobial effect on this organism.[83] Combination therapy with retinoids, BP, and topical antibiotics is commonly used and more effective than when any single agent is used alone.[82] Salicylic acid has comedolytic properties but is less potent than topical retinoids.[82]

Systemic Antibiotics

For patients with moderate and severe acne and inflammatory acne resistant to topical therapies, systemic antibiotics are the standard of care.[82] Antibiotics suppress growth of *P acnes* and directly suppress inflammation.[83] Studies have shown that doxycycline and minocycline are more effective than tetracycline and that minocycline is superior to doxycyline in reducing *P acnes*.[82] Erythromycin is also effective but is associated with higher rates of bacterial resistance. The current guidelines recommend that the use of erythromycin should be limited to individuals in whom tetracyclines are contraindicated.[82] Patients with less severe forms should not use oral antibiotics,[82] and systemic antibiotics should not be used for longer than 6 months.[83]

Hormonal Agents

Hormonal therapy should be considered in women who have adult onset acne and a history of irregular menses, hirsutism, premenstrual flares, androgenic alopecia, or who have failed standard therapy.[83] Several oral contraceptives have been approved by the FDA for the management of acne (see **Box 1**). Studies suggest other estrogen-containing OCPs may be equally effective[82] (see **Box 1**). Spironolactone (50–200 mg/d), and flutamide, two types of oral antiandrogen medications, are also effective. Spironolactone may rarely cause hyperkalemia and flutamide may cause liver toxicity.[82] Short courses of corticosteroids may be used preceding, or in conjunction with, oral retinoids in particularly extreme clinical situations.[82,83]

Isotretinoin

Oral isotretinoin is approved for the treatment of severe recalcitrant nodular acne.[82] It may also be used for patients with less severe acne who are resistant to treatment or at risk for physical or psychological scarring.[82,83] Oral isotretinoin is a potent teratogen and may be associated with the development of mood disorders, depression, suicidal ideation, hepatotoxicity, hypertriglyceridemia, and rarely pseudotumor cerebri. Because of these side effects (particularly the teratogenic effect of isotretinoin), the FDA has approved a new risk management program.[82] The iPLEDGE program requires adequate contraception counseling and women to take birth control 1 month before, during, and 1 month after isotretinoin therapy; pregnancy tests must be done before, during, and after treatment.[82] It is the only therapeutic agent that can produce prolonged remissions.

PHYSICAL TREATMENTS

Several physical treatments may be used for eradication of acne lesions, including intralesional steroids, acne surgery, laser and light source treatments, and photodynamic therapy (PDT).

Intralesional steroids are effective for individual acne nodules and cysts. Injection with triamcinolone (2.5–5 mg/mL) has been associated with a reduction in inflammation, rapid involution, and overall improvement.[85,86] Local atrophy is an associated side effect of treatment. Acne surgery includes the use of several surgical methods for active acne lesions and postscarring acne. These surgical procedures include comedo removal, chemical peels, laser and light therapy, and cryotherapy. For active lesions, comedone extraction and superficial chemical peels may be used only as an adjunct to pharmacologic treatments.[86]

Light and laser treatment has recently emerged as a therapeutic option for patients with inflammatory acne. Natural and artificial ultraviolet light is associated with an improvement of inflammatory acne lesions [87] through a mechanism known as the photodynamic response. P acnes proliferation causes the production of protoporphyrin IX (PpIX) and coproporphyrin III within the sebaceous gland.[88] The peak absorption of PpIX occurs at the blue (415 nm) and red (630 nm) light range of the visible light spectrum. Absorption of this light energy leads to local and selective destruction of the inflammatory acne lesion.[88]

Since this discovery, many light sources have been developed, one of which is the blue light. Blue light sources have been shown to destroy P acnes and have been approved by the FDA to treat mild-to-moderate inflammatory acne.[88] Narrow band blue light (420 nm) not only exerts a phototoxic effect on heme metabolism of P acnes but also has been shown to have antiinflammatory effects on keratinocytes, thereby modulating the inflammatory process of acne vulgaris.[89]

The combination of 20% 5-aminolevulinic acid (ALA) with PDT is a novel treatment for acne vulgaris. ALA is an exogenous PDT reaction that may be combined with various light sources including blue light and intense pulse light. Although ALA is considered off-label use for the treatment of acne vulgaris, several trials have shown improvement of moderate-to-severe inflammatory acne vulgaris.[90–95] Incubation with ALA and laser sources varies across studies. Reported side effects include postinflammatory hyperpigmentation, superficial peeling, and crusting.[90]

SUMMARY

Acne is the most common disease of the skin. It affects 85% of teenagers, 42.5% of men, and 50.9% of women between the ages of 20 and 30 years.[96,97] The role of hormones, particularly as a trigger of sebum production and sebaceous growth and differentiation, is well known. Excess production of hormones, specifically androgens, GH, IGF-1, insulin, CRH, and glucocorticoids, is associated with increased rates of acne development.

Acne may be a feature in many endocrine disorders, including polycystic ovary disease, Cushing syndrome, CAH, androgen-secreting tumors, and acromegaly. Other nonendocrine diseases associated with acne include Apert syndrome, SAPHO syndrome, Behçet syndrome and PAPA syndrome.

Acne medicamentosa is the development of acne vulgaris or an acneiform eruption with the use of certain medications. These medications include testosterone, progesterone, steroids, lithium, phenytoin, isoniazid, vitamins B_2, B_6, and B_{12}, halogens, and epidermal growth factor inhibitors. Management of acne medicamentosa includes standard acne therapy. Discontinuation of the offending drug may be necessary in recalcitrant cases.

Basic therapeutic interventions for acne include topical therapy, systemic antibiotics, hormonal agents, isotretinoin, and physical treatments. Generally, the severity of acne lesions determines the type of acne regimen necessary. The emergence of drug-resistant *P acnes* and adverse side effects are current limitations to effective acne management.

REFERENCES

1. Stern RS. The prevalence of acne based on physical examination. J Am Acad Dermatol 1992;26(6):931–5.
2. Thiboutot D. Acne: hormonal concepts and therapy. Clin Dermatol 2004;22(5): 419–28.
3. Cassidy DM, Lee CM, Laker MF, et al. Lipogenesis in isolated human sebaceous glands. FEBS Lett 1986;200(1):173–6.
4. Proksch E, Feingold KR, Elias PM. Epidermal HMG CoA reductase activity in essential fatty acid deficiency: barrier requirements rather than eicosanoid generation regulate cholesterol synthesis. J Invest Dermatol 1992;99:216–20.
5. Smythe CD, Greenall M, Kealey T. The activity of HMG-CoA reductase and acetyl-CoA carboxylase in human apocrine sweat glands, sebaceous glands and hair follicles is regulated by phosphorylation and by exogenous cholesterol. J Invest Dermatol 1998;111(1):139–48.
6. Toyoda M, Morohashi M. Pathogenesis of acne. Med Electron Microsc 2001; 34(1):29–40.
7. Oberemok SS, Shalita AR. Acne vulgaris I: pathogenesis and diagnosis. Cutis 2002;70(2):101–5.
8. Choudhry R, Hodgins MB, Van der Kwast TH, et al. Localization of androgen receptors in human skin by immunohistochemistry: implications for the hormonal regulation of hair growth, sebaceous glands and sweat glands. J Endocrinol 1992;133(3):467–75.
9. Liang T, Hoyer S, Yu R, et al. Immunocytochemical localization of androgen receptors in human skin using monoclonal antibodies against the androgen receptor. J Invest Dermatol 1993;100(5):663–6.
10. Zouboulis C. Acne and sebaceous gland function. Clin Dermatol 2004;22(5): 360–6.
11. Rosenfield RL, Deplweski D, Kentsis A, et al. Mechanisms of androgen induction of sebocyte differentiation. Dermatology 1998;196(1):43–6.
12. Brun RP, Tontonoz P, Forman BM, et al. Differential activation of adipogenesis by multiple PPAR isoforms. Genes Dev 1996;10(8):974–84.
13. Strauss J, Pochi PE. Effect of cyclic progestin-estrogen therapy on sebum and acne in women. JAMA 1964;190(9):815–9.
14. Zouboulis CC, Schagen S, Alestas T. The sebocyte culture: a model to study the pathophysiology of the sebaceous gland in sebostasis, seborrhea and acne. Arch Dermatol Res 2008;300(8):397–413.
15. Deplewski D, Rosenfield RL. Role of hormones in pilosebaceous unit development. Endocr Rev 2000;21(4):363–92.

16. Ozegovic B, Milkovic S. Effects of adrenocorticotrophic hormone, growth hormone, prolactin, adrenalectomy and corticoids upon weight, protein and nucleic acid content of the female rat preputial glands. Endocrinology 1972;90(4): 903–8.

17. Ebling FJ, Ebling E, Randall V, et al. The sebotrophic action of growth hormone (BGH) in the rat. Br J Dermatol 1975;92(3):325–32.

18. Deplewski D, Rosenfield RL. Growth hormone and insulin-like growth factors have different effects on sebaceous cell growth and differentiation. Endocrinology 1999;140(9):4089–94.

19. Vora S, Ovhal A, Jerajani H, et al. Correlation of facial sebum to serum insulin-like growth factor-1 in patients with acne. Br J Dermatol 2008;159(4):979–95.

20. Smith RN, Mann NJ, Braue A, et al. The effect of high-protein, low glycemic-load diet versus a conventional, high glycemic-load diet on biochemical parameters associated with acne vulgaris: a randomized, investigator-masked, controlled trial. J Am Acad Dermatol 2007;57(2):247–56.

21. Willis D, Mason H, Gilling-Smith C, et al. Modulation by insulin of follicle-stimulating and luteinizing hormone action in human granulosa cells of normal and polycystic ovaries. J Clin Endocrinol Metab 1996;81(1):302–9.

22. Kristiansen S, Endoh A, Casson P, et al. Induction of steroidogenic enzyme genes by insulin and IGF-I in cultured adult human adrenocortical cells. Steroids 1997;62(2):258–65.

23. Smith RN, Braue A, Varigos GA, et al. The effect of a low glycemic load diet on acne vulgaris and the fatty acid composition of skin surface triglycerides. J Dermatol Sci 2008;50(1):41–52.

24. Smith TM, Gilliland K, Clawson GA, et al. IGF-1 induces SREBP-1 expression and lipogenesis in SEB-1 sebocytes via activation of the phosphoinositide 3-kinase/Akt pathway. J Invest Dermatol 2008;128(5):1286–93.

25. Kaymak Y, Adisen E, Itler N, et al. Dietary glycemic index and glucose, insulin, insulin-like growth factor-1, insulin-like growth factor binding protein 3, and leptin levels in patients with acne. J Am Acad Dermatol 2007;57(5):819–23.

26. Zouboulis CC, Baron JM, Bohm M, et al. Frontiers in sebaceous gland biology and pathology. Exp Dermatol 2008;17(6):542–51.

27. Zouboulis CC, Seltmann H, Hiroi N, et al. Corticotropin-releasing hormone: an autocrine hormone that promotes lipogenesis in human sebocytes. Proc Natl Acad Sci U S A 2002;14(99):7148–53.

28. Ganceviciene R, Marciukaitiene I, Graziene V, et al. New accents in the pathogenesis of acne vulgaris. Acta Medica Lituanica 2006;13:83–7.

29. Shome B, Saffran M. Peptides of the hypothalamus. J Neurochem 1966;13(5): 433–48.

30. Bohm M, Schiller M, Stander S, et al. Evidence of expression of melanocortin-1 receptor in human sebocytes in vitro and in situ. J Invest Dermatol 2002;118(3): 533–9.

31. Ganceviciene R, Graziene V, Bohm M, et al. Increased in situ expression of melanocortin-1 receptor in sebaceous glands of lesional skin of patients with acne vulgaris. Exp Dermatol 2007;16(7):547–52.

32. Shibata M, Katsuyama M, Onodera T, et al. Glucocorticoids enhance toll-like receptor 2 expression in human keratinocytes stimulated with Priopionibacterium acnes or proinflammatory cytokines. J Invest Dermatol 2009;129(2): 375–82.

33. Lowenstein EJ. Diagnosis and management of the dermatologic manifestations of the polycystic ovary syndrome. Dermatol Ther 2006;19(4):210–23.

34. Robboy SJ, Kurman RJ, Merino MJ. The female reproductive system. In: Rubin E, Gorstein F, Rubin R, et al, editors. Rubin's pathology: clinicopathologic foundations of medicine. 4th edition. Philadelphia: Lippincott Williams and Wilkins; 2005. p. 967–9.

35. Cusan L, Dupont A, Gomez JL, et al. Comparison of flutamide and spironolactone in the treatment of hirsutism: a randomized controlled trial. Fertil Steril 1994;61(2):281–7.

36. Liepa GU, Sengupta A, Karsies D. Polycystic ovary syndrome (PCOS) and other androgen excess-related conditions: can changes in dietary intake make a difference? Nutr Clin Pract 2008;23(1):63–71.

37. Tan S, Hahn S, Benson S, et al. Metformin improves polycystic ovary syndrome symptoms irrespective of pre-treatment insulin resistance. Eur J Endocrinol 2007;157(5):669–76.

38. Braverman IM. Endocrine and metabolic disorders. In: Braverman IM, editor. Skin signs of systemic disease. Philadelphia: WB Saunders Company; 1998. p. 452–7.

39. Lin-Su K, Nimkarn S, New M. Congenital adrenal hyperplasia in adolescents: diagnosis and management. Ann N Y Acad Sci 2008;1135:95–8.

40. Merke DP, Bornstein SR. Congenital adrenal hyperplasia. Lancet 2005; 365(9477):2125–36.

41. Thalmann S, Meier CA. Acne and 'mild' adrenal hyperplasia. Dermatology 2006; 213(4):277–8.

42. Cordera F, Grant C, van Heerden J, et al. Androgen-secreting adrenal tumors. Surgery 2003;134(6):874–80.

43. Placzek M, Arnold B, Schmidt H, et al. Elevated 17-hydroxyprogesterone serum values in male patients with acne. J Am Acad Dermatol 2005;53(6):955–8.

44. Degitz K, Placzek M, Arnold B, et al. Congenital adrenal hyperplasia and acne in male patients. Br J Dermatol 2003;148(6):1263–6.

45. New MI. Extensive clinical experience: nonclassical 21-hydroxylase deficiency. J Clin Endrocrinol Metab 2006;91(11):4205–14.

46. New M. Nonclassical 21-hydroxylase deficiency. J Clin Endocrinol Metab 2006; 91(11);4205–14, Erratum in: J Clin Endocrinol Metab 2007;92(1):142.

47. D'Alva CB, Abiven-Lepage G, Viallon V, et al. Sex steroids in androgen-secreting adrenocortical tumors: clinical and hormonal features in comparison with non-tumor causes of androgen excess. Eur J Endocrinol 2008;159(5): 641–7.

48. Carmina E, Rosato F, Janni A, et al. Extensive clinical experience: relative prevalence of different androgen excess disorders in 950 women referred because of clinical hyperandrogenism. J Clin Endocrinol Metab 2006;91(1):2–6.

49. Strauss J, Thioboutut D. Acne vulgaris and acneiform eruptions. In: Freedberg I, Eisen A, Wolf K, et al, editors. Fitzpatrick's dermatology in general medicine. 5th edition. New York: McGraw-Hill; 1999. p. 769–83.

50. Chalmers RJ, Ead RD, Beck MH. Acne vulgaris and hidradentitis suppurativa as presenting features of acromegaly (Clin Res Ed). Br Med J 1983;287(6402): 1346–7.

51. Rizvi AA. Some clues and pitfalls in the diagnosis of acromegaly. Endocr Pract 2004;10(4):348–52.

52. Benjamin LT, Trowers AB, Schachner LA. Successful acne management in Apert syndrome twins. Pediatr Dermatol 2005;22(6):561–5.

53. DeGiovanni CV, Jong C, Woollons A. What syndrome is this? Apert syndrome. Pediatr Dermatol 2007;24(2):186–8.

54. Dolenc-Voljc M, Finzgar-Perme M. Successful isotretinoin treatment of acne in a patient with Apert syndrome. Acta Derm Venereol 2008;88(5):534–5.

55. Hsieh T, Ho N. Resolution of acne following therapy with an oral contraceptive in a patient with Apert syndrome. J Am Acad Dermatol 2005;53(1):173–4.

56. Solomon LM, Cohen MM, Pruzansky S. Pilosebaceous abnormalities in Apert type acrocephalosyndactyly. Birth Defects Orig Artic Ser 1971;7(8):193–5.

57. Henderson CA, Knaggs H, Clark A, et al. Apert's syndrome and androgen receptor staining of the basal cells of sebaceous glands. Br J Dermatol 1995;132(1):139–43.

58. Melnik B, Schmitz G. FGFR2 signaling and the pathogenesis of acne. J Dtsch Dermatol Ges 2008;6(9):721–8.

59. Utumi ER, Olveira Sales MA, Shinohara EH, et al. SAPHO syndrome with temporomandibular joint ankylosis: clinical, radiological, histopathological, and therapeutical correlations. Oral Surg Oral Med Oral Pathol Oral Radiol Endod 2008;105(3):e67–72.

60. Poindexter G, Martinez S, Roubey RA, et al. Synovitis-acne-pustulosis-hyperostosis-osteitis syndrome: a dermatologist's diagnostic dilemma. J Am Acad Dermatol 2008;59(2 Suppl 1):S53–4.

61. Iqbal M, Kolodney MS. Acne fulminans with synovitis-acne-pustulosis-hyperostosis-osteitis (SAPHO) syndrome treated with infliximab. J Am Acad Dermatol 2005;52(5 Suppl 1):S118–20.

62. Yazici H, Fresko I, Yurdakul S. Behçet's syndrome: disease manifestations, management, and advances in treatment. Nat Clin Pract Rheumatol 2007;3(3):148–55.

63. Hatemi G, Fresko I, Tascilar K, et al. Increased enthesopathy among Behçet's syndrome patients with acne and arthritis: an ultrasonography study. Arthritis Rheum 2008;58(5):1539–45.

64. Sfikakis PP, Markomichelakis N, Alpsoy E, et al. Anti-TNF therapy in the management of Behçet's disease-review and basis for recommendations. Rheumatology 2007;46(5):736–41.

65. Stichweh DS, Punaro M, Pascual V. Dramatic improvement of pyoderma gangrenosum with infliximab in a patient with PAPA syndrome. Pediatr Dermatol 2005;22(3):262–5.

66. Wise CA, Gillum JD, Seidman CE, et al. Mutations in CD2BP1 disrupt binding to PTP PEST and are responsible for PAPA syndrome, an autoinflammatory disorder. Hum Mol Genet 2002;11(8):961–9.

67. Fitzpatrick JE, Aeling JL. Acne and acneiform eruptions. In: James EF, John LA, editors. Dermatology secrets in color. 2nd edition. Philadelphia: Elsevier; 2005. p. 146–54.

68. Chan HH, Wing Y, Su R, et al. A control study of the cutaneous side effects of chronic lithium therapy. J Affect Disord 2000;57(1–3):107–13.

69. Webster GF. Pustular drug eruptions. Clin Dermatol 1993;11(4):541–3.

70. Gupta AK, Knowles SR, Gupta MA, et al. Lithium therapy associated with hidradenitis suppurativa: case report and a review of the dermatologic side effects of lithium. J Am Acad Dermatol 1995;32(2 Pt 2):382–6.

71. Yeung CK, Chan HH. Cutaneous adverse effects of lithium; epidemiology and management. Am J Clin Dermatol 2004;5(1):3–8.

72. Jacobsen NW, Halling-Sorensen B, Birkved FK. Inhibition of human aromatase complex (CYP19) by antiepileptic drugs. Toxicol In Vitro 2008;22(1):146–53.

73. Scheinfeld N. Phenytoin in cutaneous medicine: its uses, mechanisms, and side effects. Dermatol Online J 2003;9(3):6.
74. Scheinfeld N. Impact of phenytoin therapy on the skin and skin disease. Expert Opin Drug Saf 2004;3(6):655–65.
75. Jansen T, Romiti R, Kreuter A, et al. Rosacea fulminans triggered by high-dose vitamin B6 and B12. J Eur Acad Dermatol Venereol 2001;15(5):484–5.
76. Dupre A, Albarel N, Bonafe JL, et al. Vitamin B-12 induced acne. Cutis 1979; 24(2):210–1.
77. Braun-Falco O, Lincke H. The problem of vitamin B6/B12 acne. A contribution on acne medicamentosa. MMW Munch Med Wochenschr 1976;118(6):155–60.
78. Sherertz EF. Acneiform eruption due to "megadose" vitamins B6 and B12. Cutis 1991;48(2):119–20.
79. Doebelin B, Ly A, Allombert C, et al. [Dermatological side effects of epidermal growth factor receptor inhibitors]. Presse Med 2008;37(3 Pt 2):485–9 [in French].
80. Hannoud S, Rixe O, Bloch J, et al. Skin signs associated with epidermal growth factor inhibitors. Acta Derm Venereol 2006;133(3):239–42.
81. Duvic M. EGFR inhibitor-associated acneiform folliculitis: assessment and management. Am J Clin Dermatol 2008;9(5):285–94.
82. Strauss JS, Krowchuk DP, Leyden JJ, et al. Guidelines of care for acne vulgaris management. J Am Acad Dermatol 2007;56(4):651–63.
83. Oberemok SS, Shalita AR. Acne vulgaris, II: treatment. Cutis 2002;70(2):111–6.
84. Tenaud I, Khammari A, Dreno B. In vitro modulation of TLR2, CD1d and IL-10 by adapalene on normal human skin and acne inflammatory lesions. Exp Dermatol 2007;16(6):500–6.
85. Levine RM, Rasmussen JE. Intralesional corticosteroids in the treatment of nodulocystic acne. Arch Dermatol 1983;119(6):480–1.
86. Khunger N. Standard guidelines for acne surgery. Indian J Dermatol Venereol Leprol 2008;74(Suppl):S28–36.
87. Sigurdsson V, Knulst AC, van Weelden H. Phototherapy of acne vulgaris with visible light. Dermatology 1997;194(3):256–60.
88. Gold MH. Acne and PDT: new techniques with laser and light sources. Lasers Med Sci 2007;22(2):67–72.
89. Shnitkind E, Yaping E, Geen S, et al. Anti-inflammatory properties of narrow-band blue light. J Drugs Dermatol 2006;5(7):605–10.
90. Hongcharu W, Taylor CR, Chang Y, et al. Topical ALA-photodynamic therapy for the treatment of acne vulgaris. J Invest Dermatol 2000;115(2):183–92.
91. Itoh Y, Ninomiya Y, Tajima S, et al. Photodynamic therapy of acne vulgaris with topical 5-aminolevulinic acid. Arch Dermatol 2000;136(9):1093–5.
92. Gold MH. A multi-center study of photodynamic therapy in the treatment of moderate to severe inflammatory acne vulgaris with topical 20% 5-aminolevulinic acid and a new intense pulsed light source. J Am Acad Dermatol 2004; 50(3 Suppl 1):14.
93. Taub AF. Photodynamic therapy for the treatment of acne: a pilot study. J Drugs Dermatol 2004;3(6 Suppl):S10–4.
94. Santos MA, Belo VG, Santos G. Effectiveness of photodynamic therapy with topical 5-aminolevulinic acid and intense pulsed light versus intense pulsed light alone in the treatment of acne vulgaris: a comparative study. Dermatol Surg 2005;31(8 Pt 1):910–5.
95. Rojanamatin J, Choawawanich P. Treatment of inflammatory facial acne vulgaris with intense pulsed light (IPL) and short contact of topical 5-aminolevulinic acid: a pilot study. Dermatol Surg 2006;32(8):991–7.

96. Johnson ML, Johnson KG, Engel A. Prevalence, morbidity and cost of dermatologic diseases. J Am Acad Dermatol 1984;11(5 Pt 2):930–6.
97. Collier CN, Harper JC, Cafardi JA, et al. The prevalence of acne in adults 20 years and older. J Am Acad Dermatol 2008;58(1):56–9.
98. Camacho-Martinez FM. Hair, nails, and mucous membranes. In: Bolognia JL, Jorizzo JL, Rapini RP, et al, editors. Dermatology. 2nd edition. vol. 1. Philadelphia: Mosby Elsevier; 2008. p. 1017.
99. Zaenglein AL, Thioboutot DM. Acne vulgaris. In: Bolognia JL, Jorizzo JL, Rapini RP, et al, editors. Dermatology. 2nd edition. vol. 1. Philadelphia: Mosby Elsevier; 2008. p. 536.
100. Aron DC, Findling JW, Tyrrell JB. Glucocorticoids and adrenal androgens. In: Greenspan FS, Gardner DG, editors. Basic & clinical endocrinology. 7th edition. New York: Lange Medical Books/McGraw-Hill; 2004. p. 362–413.
101. Orth DN, Kovacs WJ. The adrenal cortex. In: Wilson JD, Foster DW, Kronenberg HM, et al, editors. Williams textbook of endocrinology. 9th edition. Philadelphia: WB Saunders Company; 1998. p. 517–664.

Rosacea

Guy F. Webster, MD, PhD[a,b,*]

KEYWORDS

• Rosacea • Acne • Rhinophyma • Blush • Keratosis pilaris

Rosacea, a common disease in adults, has an extremely variable presentation. Severity is also highly variable and, to some degree, the location of mild end of the rosacea spectrum is in the eye of the beholder. Rosacea has been noted since at least the Middle Ages. The red-faced drunk (**Fig. 1**) and the swollen nose of the self-indulgent are images from Shakespeare and Chaucer that have been used in modern political cartoons as well. This association with alcohol and excess is unfortunate since most patients are neither alcoholic nor dissipated.

EPIDEMIOLOGY

Rosacea is thought of as a disease of the fair-skinned, but this is not exclusively the case. Patients of any ethnic group may be afflicted with the disease. Rosacea may be seen in childhood or extreme old age, but typically is at its worst in the 30s through 50s.[1,2] Exact incidence data are lacking because of difficulty in defining when the disease begins. At what point does a patient's rosy cheeks become the vascular manifestation of rosacea? A Swedish study reported an incidence of 10%, which seems to be a reasonable number.[3] Data on the incidence in various racial and ethnic groups are generally lacking, but it is reasonable to say that the disease (and its detection) is highest in the lighter-skinned.

ETIOLOGY

Largely because scientists have only recently had the intellectual tools to explain rosacea, the causes of the disease, despite its long history, are only beginning to be understood (**Fig. 2**).

There are clear neurological influences in rosacea. Rosacea patients give a history of easy blushing and flushing and, with time, report a general reddening of the complexion. Foods and medications that induce facial vasodilatation seem to speed the onset of rosacea. Wilkin[4–6] has shown that the vasodilation of rosacea patients is greater and more persistent than that seen in normal volunteers. It had long been assumed that caffeine is the cause of blushing in spite of the fact that it is

[a] Department of Dermatology, Jefferson Medical College, Philadelphia, PA, USA
[b] Webster Dermatology, Suite 10, 740 Yorklyn Road, Hockessin, DE 19707, USA
* Corresponding author.
E-mail address: guywebster@yahoo.com

Med Clin N Am 93 (2009) 1183–1194
doi:10.1016/j.mcna.2009.08.007
0025-7125/09/$ – see front matter © 2009 Elsevier Inc. All rights reserved.

medical.theclinics.com

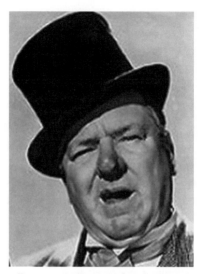

Fig. 1. Note the red and swollen nose indicative of early rhinophyma.

a vasoconstrictor. It turns out, however, that the temperature of the coffee or tea, rather than the caffeine, that causes a blush. Wilkin has also clearly shown that thermal stimuli cause food-induced flushing in most cases. Although rosacea is not commonly thought of as a neurological disease, it must be remembered that blushing is a neurally mediated function and that rosacea thus has in part a neurological basis. Indeed, studies report an increased incidence of rosacea in Parkinsonism.[7]

The reason why vasodilation promotes rosacea is unclear. It has been proposed that minute amounts of plasma are extravasated by the blush, which then induces an inflammatory response that grows with repeated episodes of vasodilation, resulting in chronic vasodilation and smoldering inflammation analogous to the dermatitis seen with chronic leg edema.[5]

Patients with rosacea also have a defective skin barrier and may be hyperirritable. Patients often complain of stinging and burning from cosmetics and medications. Some data corroborate this. Dirschka and colleagues[8] demonstrated increased transepidermal water loss in the skin of perioral dermatitis patients, but not those with malar rosacea. Laquieze and coworkers[9] found a defective barrier as measured by transepidermal water loss, lactic acid stinging, and electrical capacitance, which was corrected by treatment of the disease and moisturization.

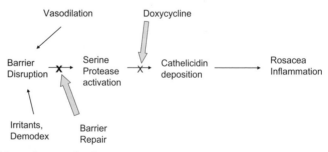

Fig. 2. Possible pathogenesis of rosacea.

Cathelicidin and serine protease activity is also clearly involved in the pathogenesis of rosacea and may be central to the disease. Gallo and colleagues[10] have demonstrated that elevated epidermal serine protease activity occurs in rosacea and causes the deposition of cathelicidin-derived peptides in the skin. These peptides have the ability to cause inflammation when injected in the skin.

Voegeli and colleagues[11] showed that defective barriers have elevations in serine proteases that normalize when the barrier is corrected. This shows a possible link between barrier function and inflammation.

In the past 15 or so years, an apparent association between *Helicobacter pylori* and rosacea has been reported. Patients treated for gastritis were found to have reduced severity of their inflammatory rosacea. Also, an increased incidence of *H pylori* was reported among rosacea patients.[12–14] Subsequent studies have clearly demonstrated that the association is merely the coincidence of two common conditions that happen to respond to the same medications. Schneider and colleagues and Sharma and colleagues[15–19] demonstrated that seroreactivity to helicobacter is no greater in rosacea patients. Similarly, endoscopic biopsy of rosacea patients revealed an identical prevalence of helicobacter infection with nonrosacea patients.

Demodex folliculorum, a mite that lives within the lumen of the sebaceous follicles of the head, has been implicated in rosacea for decades, but evidence of a link has been largely circumstantial. Lacey and colleagues[20] have demonstrated in vitro that *D folliculorum* has antigens that react with sera from rosacea patients and is capable of stimulating mononuclear cells to proliferate. *D folliculorum* mites reside predominantly in the follicles in the center of the face and more such mites are seen in rosacea patients than normals.[20–22] Follicles with *D folliculorum* in residence may be shown to have a surrounding inflammatory response.[23] Problems with the theory include difficulty in sampling follicular contents in a rigorous manner and the fact that most rosacea medications improve the disease but do not affect the mite. Conversely, treatment with lindane does not improve rosacea in my experience. It may be that the apparently increased population of *D folliculorum* is a consequence rather than the cause of rosacea. At most it appears that *D folliculorum* may be an exacerbating factor in predisposed individuals.

Various minimally investigated factors may worsen rosacea in certain individuals. Menopausal flushing occurs in a subset of rosacea patients and occasionally responds to oral clonidine, which does not appear to be effective for flushing in nonmenopausal patients. The severe acne patient who slowly evolves into rosacea while in his 20s implies a role for *Propionibacterium acnes* hypersensitivity in some. Neurological diseases, such as parkinsonism, clearly alter facial vasoreactivity and potentiate rosacea. Occasionally, oral niacin therapy of hyperlipidemia will trigger or worsen rosacea. Use of topical steroids on the face induces rosacea. Connective tissue disease and its therapy may worsen rosacea, thereby complicating the management of both diseases. Coexistent seborrheic dermatitis often develops in individuals with rosacea and complicates its therapy. Photodamage may also contribute to rosacea.

ENDOCRINOPATHY

Rarely, patients with a neuroendocrine tumor, such as pheochromocytoma, carcinoid, or mastocytosis, will initially present with symptoms of rosacea. Clues to the presence of these syndromes include rapid onset of the rosacea, accompanying bouts of tachycardia, hypertension, sweats, hot flashes, pruritus, or gastrointestinal symptoms, particularly diarrhea (**Box 1**).

Box 1
Suggested workup when a systemic rosacea stimulus is suspected
Careful history and examination
Twenty-four-hour urine for 5-hydroxyindolencetic acid, blood serotonin level
Twenty-four-hour urine histamine
Plasma and urine metanephrines

CLINICAL FEATURES

The clinical presentation of rosacea is varied. There are four primary subtypes— "erythematotelangiectatic" (ie, vascular), inflammatory, phymatous, and ocular— and several variants—granulomatous, pyoderma faciale, and perioral dermatitis.[24]

Vascular Rosacea

The earliest possible clinical stage of vascular rosacea is a recurrent blush. With time, the blush lasts longer and eventually is fixed. Telangiectasia begin to form initially in the alae nasi and then appear on the nose and cheeks. In some individuals, larger spider angiomata develop. It appears that the size of telangiectasia is determined to some degree by the amount of sun damage that has occurred. The most photoatrophic skin often has the most impressive blood vessels.

Whether a healthy blush warrants a diagnosis of rosacea is rightfully a matter of controversy. In the view of many experts, rosacea does not begin at least until erythema is constant. Still, this threshold may be too low since it would brand the populations of whole countries with a diagnosis of rosacea.

Edema is sometimes a clinical feature of rosacea. With recurrent vasodilation, patients sense a feeling of fullness of the cheeks and the physician can often discern a subtle induration of the cheeks. This typically responds slowly to tetracyclines. Plewig and colleagues and others[25–30] have noted a variant of rosacea in which a persistent woody induration develops and is responsive to isotretinoin.

Sebaceous Hyperplasia

Overgrowth of sebaceous glands may be a prominent feature in some rosacea patients. Rhinophyma (**Fig. 3**), the nasal sebaceous hyperplasia, is clearly linked to the disease. Initially, the skin of the nose becomes slightly swollen and smoother. Pores become more apparent as keratinous debris accumulate and glandular tissue swells. Gradually, a lumpy surface develops. Histologically, the process is initially one of sebaceous overgrowth. As rhinophyma becomes more established, accompanying fibrosis develops. Patients should be made aware that rhinophyma is uncommon in rosacea and that progression to rhinophyma is not the norm.

Isolated hyperplastic sebaceous glands are commonly seen in patients with and without rosacea and a link to the process seems real but is less certain. Most common on the forehead, these lesions can also occur on the cheeks and chin.

Inflammatory Rosacea

The spectrum of inflammation in rosacea is similar to that of acne and runs from small papules and pustules to deep persistent nodules. Reflecting the vasoreactivity of the individuals, rosacea papules are a deeper red than similar ones in acne. Also in distinction to acne, rosacea lesions are not centered on a comedo or a follicle and follicular

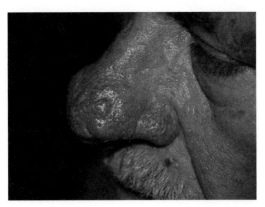

Fig. 3. Rhinophyma.

keratinization defects play no role in the process. Typically, inflammation is greatest on the central cheeks, but can also occur on the rest of the face and rarely the center of the chest. The most common lesions are small papulopustules, but large granulomatous nodules may also occur.

Ocular Rosacea

Although underappreciated by dermatologists, ocular rosacea is extremely common, with some ophthalmologic series reporting an incidence of 50% in rosacea patients. While this figure may be a bit elevated because of patient recruitment issues, it is clear that ocular rosacea is widespread. Symptoms range from a sensation of dryness or tired eyes to edema, tearing, pain, blurry vision, styes, chalazia, and corneal damage. Patients often blame contact lenses or air pollution for their problem and symptoms aren't reported to the dermatologist. Physical findings include blepharitis, meibomian impaction, styes, keratitis, and corneal neovascularization, ulceration, and even rupture.

Initially, ocular rosacea was attributed to tear film acidity, but more recent studies disprove this concept. Rather, it is thought that meibomian gland impaction leads to decreased lipid in the tear film, greater tear evaporation, and subsequent irritability of the eye.[31–34] Epithelium-derived protease activity, particularly MMP9 activity, is elevated in ocular rosacea tear fluid. In vitro studies have shown that MMP9 is inhibited by doxycycline.[35,36]

The severity of ocular rosacea is not proportional to the severity of facial disease. Patients with nodular cheek rosacea may have quiet eyes, and patients with severe blepharitis may have negligible facial inflammation. It may be helpful to ask specifically about a history of styes, which are clearly increased in rosacea. No rosacea examination is complete without evaluation of the eye.

Periorificial Dermatitis

Perioral dermatitis (**Fig. 4**) and periocular dermatitis often appear in patients with vascular rosacea but with minimal malar inflammation. Clinically, small pink papules and pustules recur over weeks to months. Various environmental sensitivities have been reported in individual patients, but a generally applicable explanation is lacking.[37] The link to rosacea is not certain, but probable. The histopathology is similar to that for rosacea.[38] The diseases occur in the same population and respond to the same medications.

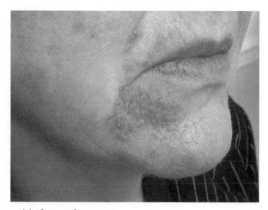

Fig. 4. Perioral dermatitis form of rosacea.

Pyoderma Facial

Eruptions of inflamed papules and yellow pustules in the centrofacial region have been termed *pyoderma faciale* (**Fig. 5**) or *rosacea fulminans*. Like periorificial dermatitis, pyoderma faciale is linked to rosacea in that it is similar histologically and responds to some of the same medications.[39,40] Patients are typically younger and are more often female. Also, the disease may begin with very little prior history of rosacea. In many cases, the patient has been treated for various infections with no success. In the past few years, I have seen pyoderma faciale in patients who were worked up for leishmaniasis and blastomycosis and in patients treated with multiple courses of intravenous antibiotics before the correct diagnosis was made.

Steroid Rosacea

Use of corticosteroids long term, whether topical or systemic, inevitably results in exacerbation of rosacea. Initially, the rosacea improves, but after prolonged use, atrophy, persistent vasodilation, and inflammatory papules develop.[41,42] The presence of rosacealike lesions on the upper lip and around the ala nasi is a clue to steroid involvement. Fluorinated and other potent steroids cause problems more quickly, but any topical (or inhaled[43]) steroid is probably capable of inducing rosacea. Often there

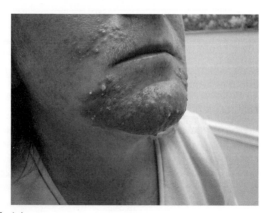

Fig. 5. Pyoderma faciale.

is no clear history of steroid usage. In these situations, the doctor must be diligent in taking a very thorough history of all of the products applied to the face. Steroids have been reported to have been surreptitiously added to many homeopathic products. Bleaching creams from outside the United States have also been reported to some-times have high-potency steroids not listed on the label. Withdrawal of the steroid is required and might as well be done abruptly; I have found that a gentle taper of steroid use is rarely effective. The flare of rosacea will be dramatic upon steroid withdrawal and can be blunted by oral therapy with prednisone, doxycycline, minocycline, or iso-tretinoin. Topical tacrolimus has also proven to be very helpful in these patients,[44] although pimecrolimus, a similar molecule has yet to be found effective in rosacea.[45]

HISTOPATHOLOGY

Histologic changes in mild forms of rosacea are subtle and often limited to vascular ectasia and mild edema. As the process advances, a perivascular and perifollicular lymphohistiocytic infiltrate and elastolysis develops. Sebaceous hyperplasia may be prominent in some patients. Comedo formation is notably lacking. The most severely inflammatory forms of disease show noncaseating epithelioid granulomas and sinus tract formation.[46]

DIFFERENTIAL DIAGNOSIS
Seborrheic Dermatitis

Seborrheic dermatitis often coexists with rosacea. Ocular rosacea is frequently mis-diagnosed as seborrheic dermatitis and thus improperly treated.

Keratosis Pilaris

Keratosis pilaris facial disease can be difficult to differentiate from rosacea at times and the two diseases may coexist. A fixed blush, especially on the lateral cheeks, with fine follicular keratotic plugs characterizes facial keratosis pilaris.

Growth Factor Receptor Inhibitor "acne"

Growth factor receptor inhibitor "acne," an acute eruption that may occur during chemotherapy, can resemble severe acne or rosacea in some patients. Timing with chemotherapy is diagnostic.

Lupus

The malar erythema of lupus can be hard to differentiate from rosacea and, indeed, many lupus patients have coexistent rosacea that flares as systemic steroids are tapered. The presence of pustules and papules or blepharitis favors a diagnosis of ro-sacea. Fine scaling, pigment change, follicular plugging and scarring, and tenderness favor lupus.

Haber Syndrome

Haber syndrome is a rare familial condition in which a permanent flush is present in the entire face beginning in childhood. Follicular plugging and scarring develops in adulthood.

Acne

Typically, acne vulgaris occurs in a younger age group and is characterized by com-edonal lesions. Patients in their 20s and 30s may have both diseases simultaneously, in which case the acne is most commonly present on the jawline of women.

Basal Cell Carcinoma

Basal cell carcinoma may be indistinguishable from sebaceous hyperplasia on occasion.

THERAPY

Rosacea can be a difficult disease to treat in part because the predisposing vasodilation is largely unresponsive to topical or systemic therapy (with the exception of corticosteroids, which are contraindicated). Avoidance of obvious vasodilators and irritants is clearly helpful in a few patients, but only rarely is sufficient. Since effective rosacea treatments have been in existence for over 30 years, there are relatively few recent large-scale studies that meet current "evidence-based" criteria.

Topical Therapy

Topical metronidazole is the major topical therapy for rosacea.[47–49] Applied once or twice daily, it is most active on inflammatory lesions and may have some effect on erythema, especially that which is perilesional. Response is not immediate; sometimes several weeks are required before a benefit is seen.

Azeleic acid cream is useful in rosacea and in one study appears to be about as effective as topical metronidazole.[50] Benzoyl peroxide preparations that are not irritating are also useful in the inflammatory forms of rosacea.[51] Topical erythromycin, clindamycin, and tetracycline appear to have little effect on rosacea. Sodium sulfacetamide is an older medication that is useful for mild rosacea and as an adjunct therapy for more severe disease.

Topical tretinoin, perhaps counterintuitively (because it is an irritant in many patients), has been reported to be helpful over the long term in rosacea patients.[52] Its effect is clearly not on follicular keratinization and may have its action on the elastolysis seen in chronic rosacea.

Oral Therapy

Tetracyclines are the most commonly prescribed oral drug for rosacea.[52–54] Their mechanism of action is primarily anti-inflammatory in rosacea, since there is usually no bacterial stimulus for the disease. The anti-inflammatory activity of this family of drugs is well described.[55–57] Tetracyclines decrease the chemotactic response of neutrophils, inhibit metalloproteinases, inhibit granuloma formation, and inhibit protein kinase C. The relative potency of the tetracyclines' inhibition of granulomas parallels their clinical activity. Of the three, tetracycline is weakest, and doxycycline and minocycline about equipotent.

Traditionally, treatment was started at a high dose, which was lowered as the disease became quiet. Once rosacea is controlled, tetracyclines can be given in surprisingly small dosages (eg, 20 mg twice daily).[58] More recently,[59] a sustained release, low-dose doxycycline has become available that is effective as initial therapy and has the advantage of being below the level of antimicrobial activity. There is justifiable concern about antibiotic overuse, the spread of resistant organisms, and the possibility that long-term rosacea treatment might exacerbate resistance. The drug is designed to be purely anti-inflammatory in that antimicrobial levels of the drug are never achieved and there is no change in the microbial flora of the skin or gastrointestinal tract, thus resistance cannot develop.

Other antibiotics are occasionally useful in rosacea. Trimethoprim/sulfamethoxazole and ciprofloxacin[60] will both improve inflammatory rosacea, but are rarely used because of cost and valid concerns regarding the generation of resistant bacterial populations. Erythromycin, penicillins, and cephalosporins are of very little use in rosacea.

Isotretinoin

The most severe forms of rosacea may require isotretinoin therapy.[52,59] Inflammatory lesions and particularly refractory nodules typically respond well to 0.25 to 1 mg/kg isotretinoin. Unfortunately, a lasting response, such as is seen in acne, does not occur frequently, and patients may require long-term maintenance therapy with oral tetracyclines. The mechanism by which isotretinoin is effective is unclear because its main mode of action in acne—inhibition of the sebaceous gland—would appear to not be operative in inflammatory rosacea. Isotretinoin is also helpful in rhinophyma. Results are best if treatment is begun before significant fibrosis has developed.

Surgical Treatments

Telangiectasia and persistent erythema are effectively treated with intense pulsed light units or the pulsed dye laser.[61,62] Lasting remissions of vascular rosacea are sometimes achieved. Electrocoagulation of telangiectasia is also effective, but carries a greater risk of scarring. Carbon dioxide laser or hot loop recontouring is the only method of improving fibrotic rhinophyma.

REFERENCES

1. Marks R. Rosacea, flushing and perioral dermatitis. In: Rook R, editor. Textbook of dermatology; p. 1851–63.
2. Savin J, Alexander S, Marks R. A rosacea-like eruption of children. Br J Dermatol 1972;82:425–8.
3. Berg M, Liden S. An epidemiological study of rosacea. Acta Derm Venereol 1989; 69:419–23.
4. Wilkin JK. Rosacea [review]. Int J Dermatol 1983;22:393–400.
5. Wilkin JK. Oral thermal-induced flushing in erythematotelangiectatic rosacea. J Invest Dermatol 1981;76:15–8.
6. Wilkin JK. Rosacea. Pathophysiology and treatment. Arch Dermatol 1994;130: 359–62.
7. Fischer M, Gemende I, Marsch WC, et al. Skin function and skin disorders in Parkinson's disease. J Neural Transm 2001;108:205–13.
8. Dirschka T, Tronnier H, Folster-Holst R. Epithelial barrier function and atopic diathesis in rosacea and perioral dermatitis. Br J Dermatol 2004;150:1136–41.
9. Laquieze S, Czernielewski J, Baltas E. Beneficial use of cetaphil moisturizing cream as part of a daily skin care regimen for individuals with rosacea. J Dermatolog Treat 2007;18:158–62.
10. Yamasaki K, DiNardo A, Bardan A, et al. Increased serine protease activity and cathelicidin promotes skin inflammation in rosacea. Nat Med 2007;13: 975–80.
11. Voegli R, Rawlings AV, Doppler S, et al. Increased basal transepidermal water loss leads to elevation of some but not all stratum corneum serine proteases. Int J Cosmet Sci 2008;30:435–43.
12. Rebora A, Drago F, Picciotto A. Helilcobacter pylori in patients with rosacea. Am J Gastroenterol 1994;89:1603–4.
13. Diaz C, O'Calaghan CJ, Khan A, et al. Rosacea: a cutaneous marker for Helicobacter pylori infection? Acta Derm Venereol 2003;83:282–6.

14. Utas S, Ozbakir O, Turasan A, et al. *Helicobacter pylori* eradication treatment reduces the severity of rosacea. J Am Acad Dermatol 1999;40:433–5.
15. Sharma VK, Lynn A, Kaminski M, et al. A study of the prevalence of *Helicobacter pylori* infection and other markers of upper gastrointestinal disease in patients with rosacea. Am J Gastroenterol 1998;93:220–2.
16. Schneider MA, Skinner RBJ, Rosenberg EW. Serological determination of *Helicobacter pylori* in rosacea patients [abstract]. Clin Res 1992;40:831.
17. Bamford JTM, Tilden RT, Blankush JL, et al. Effect of treatment of *Helicobacter pylori* infection on rosacea. Arch Dermatol 1999;135:659–63.
18. Wedi B, Kapp A. *Helicobacter pylori* infection in skin diseases: a critical appraisal. Am J Clin Dermatol 2002;3:273–82.
19. Leontiadis GI, Sharma VK, Howden CW. Non-gastrointestinal tract associations of *Helicobacter pylori* infection. What is the evidence? Arch Intern Med 1999;159: 925–40.
20. Lacey N, Delaney S, Kavanagh K, et al. Mite-related bacterial antigens stimulate inflammatory cells in rosacea. Br J Dermatol 157:474–81.
21. Erbagci Z, Ozgoztasi O. The significance of *Demodex folliculorum* density in rosacea. Int J Dermatol 1998;37:421–5.
22. Roihu T, Kariniemi AL. Demodex mites in rosacea. J Cutan Pathol 1998;25:550–2.
23. Wilkin J, Detmar M, Drake L, et al. Standard classification of rosacea. J Am Acad Dermatol 2002;46.
24. Jansen T, Plewig G. Rosacea: classification and treatment. J R Soc Med 1997;90: 144–50.
25. Forton F, Seys B. Density of *Demodex folliculorum* in rosacea: a case-control study using standardized skin surface biopsy. Br J Dermatol 1993;128: 650–9.
26. Bonnar E, Eustace P, Powell FC. The demodex mite population in rosacea. J Am Acad Dermatol 1994;28:443–8.
27. Forton F, Germaux MA, Rasseur B, et al. Demodicosis and rosacea: epidemiology and significance in daily dermatologic practice. J Am Acad Dermatol 2005;52:74–87.
28. Powell FC. Rosacea and the pilosebaceous follicle. Cutis 2004;74:32–4.
29. Scerri L, Saihan EM. Persistent facial swelling in a patient with rosacea. Rosacea lymphedema. Arch Dermatol 1995;131:1071–4.
30. Bernardini FP, Kersten RC, Khouri LM, et al. Chronic eyelid edema and ocular rosacea. Report of two cases. Ophthalmology 2000;107:2220–3.
31. Stone DU, Chodosh J. Ocular rosacea an update on pathogenesis and therapy. Curr Opin Ophthalmol 2004;15:499–502.
32. Browning DJ, Proia AD. Ocular rosacea. Surv Ophthalmol 1986;31:145–58.
33. Kligman AM. Ocular rosacea: current concepts and therapy. Arch Dermatol 1997; 133:89–90.
34. Sobrin L, Liu Z, Monroy DC, et al. Regulation of MMP-9 activity in human tear fluid and corneal epithelial culture supernatant. Invest Ophthalmol Vis Sci 2000;41: 1703–9.
35. Alfonso AA, Sobrin L, Monroy DC, et al. Tear fluid gelatinase B activity correlates with IL-1alpha concentration and fluorescein clearance in ocular rosacea. Invest Ophthalmol Vis Sci 1999;40:2506–12.
36. Kerr REI, Thomsom J. Perioral dermatitis. In: Freedberg I, et al, editors. Dermatology in general medicine. 4th edition, p. 735–40.
37. Ramelet AA, Delacretaz JJ. Histopathological study of perioral dermatitis. Dermatologica 1981;47:163–71.

38. Massa MC, Su WPD. Pyoderma faciale: a clinical study of twenty-nine patients. J Am Acad Dermatol 1982;6:84–91.
39. Marks VJ, Briggaman RA. Pyoderma faciale, successful treatment with isotretinoin. J Am Acad Dermatol 1987;17:1062–4.
40. Leyden JJ, Thew M, Kligman AM. Steroid rosacea. Arch Dermatol 1974;110: 619–22.
41. Martin DL, Turner ML, Williams CM. Recent onset of smooth shiny erythematous papules on the face. Steroid rosacea secondary to topical fluorinated steroid use. Arch Dermatol 1989;125:828–31.
42. Egan CA, Rallis TM, Meadows KP, et al. Rosacea induced by beclomethasone dipropionate nasal spray. Int J Dermatol 1999;38:133–4.
43. Goldman D. Tacrolimus ointment for the treatment of steroid induced rosacea, a preliminary report. J Am Acad Dermatol 2001;44:995–9.
44. Wilkin JK. Use of topical products for maintaining remission in rosacea. Arch Dermatol 1999;135:79–82.
45. Weissbacher S, Merkl J, Hildebrandt B, et al. Pimecrolimus cream for papulopustular rosacea: a randomized vehicle controlled clinical trial. Br J Dermatol 2007;156:728–32.
46. Marks R, Harcourt-Webster JN. Histopathology of rosacea. Arch Dermatol 1969; 100:686–92.
47. Dahl MV, Katz HI, Krueger GG, et al. Topical metronidazole maintains remissions of rosacea. Arch Dermatol 1998;134:679–83.
48. Neilson PG. A double blind study of 1% metronidazole cream vs. systemic oxytetracycline therapy for rosacea. Br J Dermatol 1983;109:63–5.
49. Madden S. A comparison of topical azeleic acid 20% cream and topical metronidazole 0.75% cream in the treatment of patients with papulopustular rosacea. J Am Acad Dermatol 1999;40:961–5.
50. Leyden JJ, Thiboutot D, Shalita A. Photographic review of results from a clinical study comparing benzoyl peroxide 5% clindamycin 1% topical gel with vehicle in rosacea. Cutis 2004;73:11–7.
51. Ertl GA, Levine N, Kligman AM. A comparison of the efficacy of topical tretinoin and low dose oral isotretinoin in rosacea. Arch Dermatol 1994;130:319–24.
52. Wereide K. Long term treatment of rosacea with oral tetracycline. Acta Derm Venereol 1969;49:176–9.
53. Webster GF. Treatment of rosacea. Semin Cutan Med Surg 2001;20:207–8.
54. DelRosso JQ. Systemic therapy for rosacea, focus on oral antibiotictherapy and safety. Cutis 2000;66:7–13.
55. Van Vlem B, Vanholder R, De Paepe P, et al. Immunomodulating effects of antibiotics. Infection 1996;24:275–9.
56. Ueyama Y, Misaki M, Ishihara Y, et al. Effects of antibiotics on polymorphonucleasr leukocyte chemotaxis in vitro. Br J Oral Maxillofac Surg 1994;32:96–9.
57. Webster GF, Toso SM, Hegemann LR. Inhibition of a model of in vitro granuloma formation by tetracyclines and ciprofloxacin. Involvement of protein kinase C. Arch Dermatol 1994;130:748–52.
58. Sanchez J, Somolinos AL, Almodovar PI, et al. A randomized double blind placebo controlled trial of the combine defect of doxyxycline hycalte 20 mg tablets and metronidazole 0.75% lotion in the treatment of rosacea. J Am Acad Dermatol 2005;53:791–7.
59. DelRosso JQ, Webster GF, Jackson M, et al. Two randomized phase III clinical trials evaluating anti-inflammatory dose doxycycline administered once daily for treatment of rosacea. J Am Acad Dermatol 2007;56:791–802.

60. Marsden JR, Shuster S, Neugebauer M. Response of rosacea to isotretinoin. Clin Exp Dermatol 1984;9:484–8.
61. Laughlin SA, Dudley DK. Laser therapy in the management of rosacea. J Cutan Med Surg 1998;2(Suppl 4):S4–24.
62. West TB, Alster TS. Comparison of the long pulse dye (590–595 nm) and KTP (532 nm) lasers in the treatment of facial and leg telangiectasias. Derm Surg 1998;24:510–2.

Diseases of the Hair and Nails

Shannon Harrison, MBBS, MMed, FACD[a], Wilma F. Bergfeld, MD, FAAD, FACP[a,b],*

KEYWORDS

- Telogen effluvium • Anagen effluvium • Hair shaft disorders
- Nail disorders • Hirsutism • Hypertrichosis

HAIR DISORDERS AND INTERNAL DISEASE
Telogen Effluvium

Telogen effluvium was first described by Kligman[1] in 1961 and is defined as a sudden onset of telogen hair shedding 2 to 3 months after an acute trigger or physiologic stress.[1,2] The hair shedding occurs with a delay after the trigger or stress because of the normal hair cycle. Each hair follicle individually cycles through a growth phase (anagen) for 2 to 8 years, followed by an involution phase and into the resting phase (catagen).[3,4] Telogen lasts 2 to 3 months and the hair then cycles back to anagen.[3,4] Between 50 and 150 telogen hairs are shed normally per day.[1] With each new anagen, the hair follicle remodels itself from hair stem cells in the bulge region of the follicle.[3,4] Normally, 80% to 85% of the 100,000 hair follicles on the scalp are actively growing.[1] When a trigger or stress interrupts the normal hair cycle, a group of anagen hairs simultaneously enter catagen and cycle to telogen. These hairs are shed 2 to 3 months after the stress.

A variety of triggers or stresses can precipitate telogen hair shedding. Postpartum telogen effluvium is a well-recognized cause of physiologic telogen effluvium.[1] Other triggers include surgery,[5] high fever,[1] crash dieting,[6] nutritional deficiencies,[5,7] medications,[1,5] serious illness,[1] and emotional stress.[1] Local scalp inflammation can also cause telogen hair shedding.[7,8] If the trigger resolves or is corrected, then shedding resolves over 6 months. If telogen hair shedding continues greater than 6 months, it becomes a chronic telogen effluvium. An unrecognized trigger or repetitive or sequential triggers can cause ongoing telogen hair loss.[7] Chronic diffuse telogen hair loss can also be seen with chronic renal and liver disease, such as cirrhosis[1]; nutritional

Dr Harrison was funded by the F. C. Florance Bequest administered by the Australasian College of Dermatologists for 2008.

[a] Department of Dermatology, Cleveland Clinic Foundation, 9500 Euclid Avenue/A61, Cleveland, OH 44195, USA

[b] Department of Dermatopathology, Cleveland Clinic Foundation, 9500 Euclid Avenue/A61, Cleveland, OH 44195, USA

* Corresponding author. Department of Dermatopathology, Cleveland Clinic Foundation, 9500 Euclid Avenue/A61, Cleveland, OH 44195.

E-mail address: bergfew@ccf.org (W.F. Bergfeld).

Med Clin N Am 93 (2009) 1195–1209

doi:10.1016/j.mcna.2009.08.006

medical.theclinics.com

deficiency states or malnutrition states,[7] thyroid disease,[5,7] autoimmune conditions, such as systemic lupus erythematosus,[9] temporal arteritis,[10] and dermatomyositis.[9]

Both hypothyroidism and less commonly hyperthyroidism can cause a telogen hair shed.[5,9,11] In hypothyroidism, in addition to gradually developing diffuse scalp alopecia, loss of the outer third of the eyebrows can also be seen (Hertoghe's sign).[12] Associated body hair loss may also be noted.[9] The severity of the alopecia and the thyroid disease are typically not well correlated.[5,11] The alopecia usually improves with thyroxine replacement, unless the hypothyroidism has been long-standing.[5]

Inadequate diets of calories and protein lead to a decrease in anagen hairs and an increase in telogen hairs.[13] Nutritional deficiency states, such as marasmus (protein and caloric depletion), are associated with a diffuse telogen hair loss, in addition to hair shaft changes of thinner diameter and lighter pigmentation.[9,13] Kwashiorkor (isolated protein deficiency) can lead to thin, fragile hair with darkly pigmented hair showing the "flag sign" (alternating bands of red or white).[9,13] Essential fatty acid deficiency and biotin deficiency are less common causes of telogen effluvium.[7,9]

Iron deficiency is a controversial cause of diffuse telogen hair loss. Several studies suggest that iron deficiency with or without anemia may be a trigger for telogen effluvium, but the relationship is unclear.[14,15] Treatment for iron deficiency anemia is required with iron supplementation and monitoring of levels.[15] Treating iron deficiency without anemia is debatable, but it has been recommended to maintain ferritin levels at 70 ng/mL or greater within normal limits.[15] Hair loss also can be a sign of zinc deficiency. Associated findings include dermatitis, diarrhea, and increased frequency of infections.[7,9] Zinc replacement can restore low levels and may improve hair loss.[7,9] Zinc levels should be monitored if replacement is being used. Vitamins A and D are important vitamins in cell growth. Vitamin A deficiency can occur with restricted diets and can contribute to hair loss.[7] High levels of vitamin A also can cause hair loss.[7] Vitamin D_3 in murine models showed that vitamin D_3 may play a role in hair follicle cycling.[16] Low vitamin D levels may be a hypothetical cause of hair loss.[7]

Malabsorption states, inflammatory bowel disease, and lymphoproliferative states have also been reported to cause chronic diffuse telogen hair shedding.[1] Chronic infection, such as secondary syphilis,[5] malaria,[10] and HIV-1 infection, can also be associated with chronic diffuse telogen hair loss.[9,10] Chronic diffuse telogen hair loss without recognizable triggers and with exclusion of other causes of hair loss is known as idiopathic "chronic telogen effluvium" and is not common.[17,18]

Multiple medications can cause telogen hair shedding. Retinoids, heparin, anticonvulsants, angiotensin-converting enzyme inhibitors, and androgens can all precipitate telogen hair shedding.[19] Other listed medications can be found to cause hair loss.[9,19] Hair shedding usually occurs after 3 months of starting a drug and if the drug is stopped, the shedding ceases after approximately 3 months.[19]

A thorough medical history is important to recognize the possible stresses or triggers as a cause of hair loss. Clinically, patients experience excessive telogen hair shedding with a diffuse hair thinning over the entire scalp regardless of the initial trigger (**Fig. 1**).[7] Hair pull test and hair microscopy can reveal increased telogen hairs.[9] Laboratory investigations are needed to identify possible triggers and underlying systemic disorders including anemia, iron deficiency, renal or liver disease, thyroid disease, and zinc deficiency. Histology from scalp biopsy reveals an increased number of telogen follicles without miniaturization of the scalp hair follicles.[7]

Identification and correction of the trigger or stress usually leads to the resolution of the telogen effluvium. Adequate nutrition should be encouraged and a multivitamin with a biotin and zinc supplement can promote hair regrowth (Wilma F. Bergfeld, personal communication, 2008).[7]Sequential and repetitive triggers should be

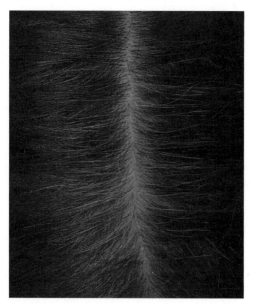

Fig. 1. Acute telogen effluvium.

recognized and treated to prevent ongoing shedding. Any identified systemic disease or infection should be treated appropriately. Off-label usage (non-FDA approved indication) of topical minoxidil 2% or 5% applied once to twice daily to the scalp may support hair regrowth.[20]

Anagen Effluvium

Acute severe stresses or triggers that interrupt hair matrix mitosis in anagen lead to a thinning and fracture of the hair shaft with anagen hair shedding.[10,21] Pigmentation of the hair shaft can also be affected.[10] Hair loss is experienced much more acutely than telogen effluvium over several days to weeks.[10] Antineoplastic agents, such as the alkylating or antimitotic agents, commonly cause anagen hair loss of the scalp, but body hair can also be lost.[19] Radiation, heavy metal, and boric acid ingestion can also trigger an anagen effluvium.[21] Radiation to the brain and busulphan treatment can cause permanent hair thinning.[19] Alopecia areata, an autoimmune condition of the hair, can also cause anagen shedding. Iatrogenic triggers are usually obvious from the medical history. Clinically, patients experience severe anagen hair shedding with a diffuse scalp alopecia because up to 80% of the hairs can be lost.[7] Hair pull test can demonstrate dystrophic, tapered anagen hairs.[21] When the trigger stops, hair growth usually can begin within weeks. In some cases with high doses of chemotherapy or radiation, the hair stem cells can be injured and hair may not regrow.[10] Observation and reassurance are required while the hair is regrowing.

Thyroid Disease

Both scalp and body hair loss may be seen with hypothyroidism.[5,9,11] Less commonly hyperthyroidism can cause a telogen effluvium.[5,9,11] Alopecia areata, an autoimmune condition of the hair causing nonscarring reversible patches of alopecia, is associated with autoimmune thyroid disease, such as Hashimoto's thyroiditis.[22] A thyroid-stimulating hormone and T4 levels can demonstrate thyroid disorders and antithyroid antibodies can help identify autoimmune associations.

Androgen Excess and Pattern Hair Loss

Hyperandrogenic states, either iatrogenic or pathologic, can cause hair loss. Pattern hair loss in men over the bitemporal scalp and crown is caused by circulating androgens and a genetic inherited susceptibility.[23,24] In women with female pattern hair loss (FPHL), there can be a genetic predisposition, but the relationship with androgen levels is uncertain.[23] In most women with FPHL, there is hair loss over the crown with retention of the frontal hair line and there is no measurable abnormality of androgen metabolism (**Fig. 2**).[23,25] Excess circulating androgens in females, such as seen with a postmenopausal androgen excess or polycystic ovarian syndrome, or an androgen-secreting tumor can cause pattern hair loss and in some cases the hair loss can resemble a male-type pattern of loss.[7,23] Associated signs of androgen excess, such as acne, hirsutism, seborrhea, and irregular menses may be present.[23] In patients with FPHL, screening blood tests for telogen effluvium should be performed in addition to an androgen screen of free or total testosterone, dihydroepiandrostene-dione sulfate, and sex-hormone binding globulin levels.[23] Scalp biopsy with horizontal and vertical sectioning shows miniaturization of the hair follicles and an increase in vellus hairs and a reduction in terminal hairs.[26]

Males with pattern hair loss may have an increased associated risk for coronary artery disease.[27] Male pattern hair loss presenting at an early age may be a marker of a carrier state for the gene for polycystic ovarian syndrome in women.[23,28] Androgen type or action medications, such as tamoxifen, anabolic steroids, and androgenic oral contraceptive pills (nortestosterone derivatives), can also cause or exacerbate a patterned hair loss.[7,19] The progestin-releasing implants can also cause similar effects.[19]

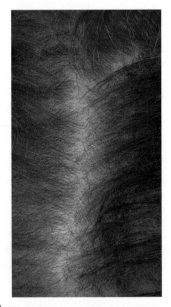

Fig. 2. Female pattern hair loss.

Treatment for male pattern hair loss involves Food and Drug Administration approved topical minoxidil 5% twice daily or the systemic agent finasteride, 1 mg daily.[23] Treatment for FPHL involves the Food and Drug Administration approved 2% minoxidil twice daily for women, although the off-label 5% minoxidil non-FDA approved for women has been shown to be better in women.[23] Antiandrogen systemic treatment for FPHL has only limited studies and is an off-label non-FDA approved use, but spironolactone in doses of 50 to 200 mg daily or one of the newer drosperinone-based oral contraceptives may improve FPHL (Wilma F. Bergfeld, personal communication, 2008).[20,23] Any antiandrogen treatment can cause feminization of the male fetus and women of child-bearing potential require effective contraception.

It should be noted that topical minoxidil can precipitate a scalp telogen hair shedding in the first 3 months of use, which usually settles.[19,20,23] Topical minoxidil can also cause facial and neck hypertrichosis, and even full body hypertrichosis if the 5% solution is used off-label in some women.[19]

Hirsutism

Hirsutism is classified as excess terminal hairs in a male-type distribution (chin, upper lip, abdomen, and chest) in women.[29] A score using the Ferrimen-Gallway scale or a modified scale can be assigned to the hirsutism after examining body areas for distribution of the hirsutism.[29,30] Hirsutism is caused by the excess action of androgens on susceptible hair follicles from overproduction of androgens from the ovaries or adrenal gland or from exogenous androgens or from increased sensitivity of the hair follicle.[29,30] Androgens cause small vellus hairs to enlarge in androgen-dependent areas into large pigmented terminal hairs, except on the scalp where the reverse occurs.[30] Hirsutism may be accompanied by other features of hyperandrogenism, such as acne, pattern hair loss, seborrhea, menstrual irregularity, and insulin resistance.

Ovarian pathologies, such as polycystic ovarian syndrome, the HAIR-AN syndrome (hyperandrogenism, insulin resistance, and acanthosis nigricans), and ovarian tumors, can cause hirsutism. Adrenal pathologies, such as a tumor, late-onset congenital adrenal hyperplasia, and Cushing syndrome, can also lead to hirsutism. Pituitary causes of hirsutism include Cushing disease, prolactinoma, and acromegaly. Exogenous androgens, such as androgenic medications in women, can also lead to hirsutism. In some women, no underlying cause for the hirsutism can be found and there are no demonstrable biochemical abnormalities; this type of hirsutism is termed "idiopathic hirsutism."[29,31] Idiopathic hirsutism may be caused by increased sensitivity of the hair follicle to circulating androgens.[29,31] If hirsutism is sudden onset and severe or accompanied by other signs of virilization (clitoromegaly, increased muscle mass, deepened voice), a tumor should be excluded.[29,30,32] Females with polycystic ovarian syndrome and the HAIR-AN syndrome are at risk for the metabolic syndrome of insulin-resistance, diabetes mellitus type II, obesity, hyperlipidemia, coronary artery disease, and possibly endometrial carcinoma.[30,32–34]

Laboratory testing should identify the etiology of the hirsutism and also include work-up for associated risks. There are no standard testing guidelines for hirsutism. The Endocrine Society, however, suggests testing for patients with hirsutism of acute onset or quick progression; moderate to severe hirsutism ferriman-gallwey (FG) score >15; or when other signs of hyperandrogenism are present of menstrual irregularity, central obesity, acanthosis nigricans, or clitoromegaly with any degree of hirsutism.[35] Testing was not recommended for women with mild hirsutism (FG scores of 8–15) because hyperandrogenemia is unable to be found in approximately half of these cases.[35] The authors test all patients with hirsutism with a basic androgen screen of a free testosterone, sex-hormone binding globulin, and dihydroepiandrostenedione sulfate level. Further information can be found in several review articles.[29,30,35,36]

Hypertrichosis

Hypertrichosis is an increase in hair growth that can be vellus, lanugo, or terminal hair type in nature in non–androgen-dependent areas of the body.[37] It can be generalized or localized. Hypertrichosis can occur as part of a hereditary syndrome or as a hereditary condition, but is more commonly acquired. Localized congenital hypertrichosis is well known in spina bifida occulta and diastematomyelia.[37] There are uncommon congenital syndromes, such as Hurler syndrome and Coffin-Siris syndrome, with generalized hypertrichosis as part of their clinical findings.[37] Acquired hypertrichosis is caused by systemic illness, such as hypothyroidism; malabsorption syndromes; central nervous system pathologies, such as head injury or multiple sclerosis; anorexia nervosa; juvenile dermatomyositis; and various porphyrias and from medications.[37] Acquired hypertrichosis lanuginosa or "malignant down" is associated with advanced internal malignancy and may appear 2 years before the malignancy presents, so patients require careful follow-up.[37]

Cyclosporin can cause hypertrichosis of the face, eyelashes, and back in 50% of patients on high-dose therapy.[19] Trichomegaly and increased pigmentation of the eyelashes have also been seen with prostaglandin F analog–containing eyedrops.[19] Multiple other medications can cause hypertrichosis including hydantoins and interferons.[19] A more detailed list of causes of hypertrichosis can be found in several references.[19,37]

Internal Conditions Associated with Hair Shaft Changes

Alterations in hair shaft pigmentation and structure can occur in several inherited metabolic syndromes and be acquired as secondary to medications. Multiple medications can cause graying or lightening of the hair including chloroquine, cyclosporine A, etretinate, and interferon-α.[19] Antineoplastics can cause increased pigmentation of the hair and curling or kinking of the hair.[19] Tamoxifen, bromocriptine, carbidopa, and verapamil can also cause hair darkening.[37] Lithium and interferon can cause hair straightening, whereas indinavir, valproic acid, and retinoids can cause hair kinking.[37]

Menkes kinky hair syndrome is a copper metabolism disorder with pili torti (hair with 180 degree twists) and short, brittle, weathered, depigmented hair.[38] Degeneration of connective tissue and cerebral tissue occurs with hypothermia, convulsions, and drowsiness seen early in life.[10,38] It is caused by a defect in the copper transporting ATPase.[38] Björnstad syndrome also has pili torti as a feature, but is associated with deafness.[10,38] Argininosuccinicaciduria is a condition characterized by a defect in the enzyme argininosuccinase and demonstrates congenital trichorrhexis nodosa (node-like abnormality of the hair shaft with loss of the cuticle) resulting in dry, dull, brittle hair.[10,38]

Trichothiodystrophy is a spectrum of findings inherited as an autosomal-recessive defect. The syndrome is characterized by brittle hair leading to short, sparse scalp hair, in addition to photosensitivity, ichthyosis, nail dystrophy, mental retardation, congenital cataracts, neutropenia, short stature, and decreased fertility.[10,38] The hair is sulfur deficient and is characterized by trichoschisis (transverse fracture) and signs of weathering on hair shaft light microscopy and a "tiger-tail appearance" with alternating light and dark bands under polarized microscopy.[10,38]

The Pohl-Pinkus mark can be seen in hairs of patients who have undergone considerable physiologic stress, such as a serious surgery or chemotherapy or severe illness.[38] The mark is a constriction of the hair shaft that coincides with a metabolic insult that decreases protein synthesis in the hair.[38] In certain nutritional deficiency states, other hair shaft abnormalities can occur. In protein and caloric malnutrition dark hair can become hypopigmented.[5] In marasmus and kwashiorkor hair shaft diameter can be reduced.[5]

Scarring alopecia

Systemic lupus erythematosus is a multisystem autoimmune condition. Systemic lupus erythematosus can cause anagen arrest and anagen hair loss, although diffuse telogen hair loss is usually more frequent.[10] The form of chronic cutaneous lupus, discoid lupus erythematosus, causes a scarring type of hair loss[39] and features of systemic lupus erythematosus are not usually present. Scarring alopecias are characterized by the loss of visible follicular openings and destruction to the regenerative stem cells in the bulge area of the hair follicle.[10] Discoid lupus erythematosus presents with areas of scarring alopecia with associated dyspigmentation, erythema, and perifollicular scale.[40] On scalp biopsy the typical interface changes, thickened basement membrane, hyperkeratosis, and follicular plugging can be seen with an associated superficial and deep inflammatory[26,40,41] infiltrative. Discoid lupus erythematosus has also presented as madarosis.[42]

Diffuse telogen hair loss and scarring alopecia can be associated with dermatomyositis.[9,10,39] Scarring alopecia can also be seen with morphea, systemic sclerosis, and chronic graft-versus-host disease.[39]

Other causes of scarring alopecias include infiltrative conditions, such as sarcoidosis, primary systemic amyloidosis, and metastases from internal malignancies.[39] Metastatic breast cancer has a preference for scalp involvement.[10] Less commonly, such infections as tuberculosis, tertiary syphilis, and leishmaniasis can cause scarring alopecia.[39] Leprosy can also cause a scarring alopecia and loss of eyebrow hair.[10]

Alopecia mucinosa is a rare condition that can present with scarring alopecia of the scalp.[38,40] On scalp biopsy, mucin deposition occurs with destruction of the outer root sheath and sebaceous glands.[26,43] Three types of alopecia mucinosa are described. Types 1 and 2 are seen in younger patients without an underlying lymphoproliferative disorder.[40] Type 3 affects older patients and is associated with an underlying lymphoproliferative malignancy.[40] Follicular T-cell mycosis fungoides can also cause a scarring alopecia when it occurs on hair-bearing areas of the scalp.[39]

NAIL DISORDERS AND INTERNAL DISEASE
Brittle Nails

Brittle nails fracture easily and onychoschizia (transverse nail splitting at the free nail edge) and onychorrhexis can be seen.[39] Many internal diseases can cause this change including hypothyroidism, hypopituitarism, acromegaly, diabetes, malnutrition, and gout.[39]

Pitting

Small round depressions in the nails caused by a defect of keratinization can be a feature of psorsiasis, alopecia areata, lichen planus, and rheumatoid arthritis (**Fig. 3**).[39,44] It can also be found in sarcoidosi, and be a normal finding.[39]

Beau Lines

Beau lines reflect an interruption to nail bed mitosis and nail production and clinically is a transverse depressed line that grows out with the nail.[39] Severe illness, high fever, or chemotherapy can cause this nail dystrophy.[44] Onychomadesis is when the nail plate

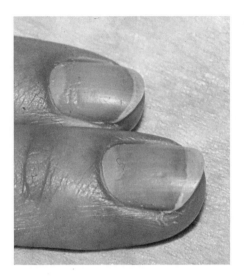

Fig. 3. Nail pitting.

detaches completely from the proximal nail fold and usually occurs when the metabolic insult is more severe.[44]

Twenty-nail Dystrophy

Increased longitudinal grooves on all nails leading to nail thinning and roughening is called "trachyonychia" (**Fig. 4**).[39] Twenty-nail dystrophy can be seen with such dermatologic conditions as psoriasis, lichen planus, eczema, and alopecia areata.[39]

Koilonychia

In koilonychia the nails are "spoon-shaped" with both a transverse and longitudinal concavity of the nail so the edges look like a spoon.[39] Koilonychia may be present in iron-deficiency anemia, but is also believed to occur in sulfur-protein deficiency and hyperthyroidism.[39] Koilonychia can also be idiopathic or familial.[39]

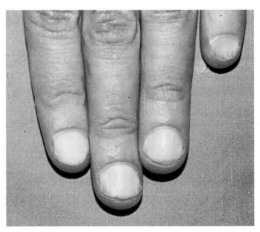

Fig. 4. Nail dystrophy.

Clubbing

Clubbed nails show an increase in the longitudinal and transverse curvature of the nail.[39] The distal region of the digit appears swollen because of hypertrophy of the soft tissue around the nail.[39] The Lovibond angle (the angle formed by the nail plate emerging from the proximal nail fold and dorsal distal phalanx) in clubbing is greater than 180 degrees compared with the normal angle, which is less than 180 degrees.[39] Although clubbing can be idiopathic or familial, it is associated with cardiac conditions, lung tumors, gastrointestinal disease, hepatic diseases, and hypertrophic osteoarthropathy.[39,44] It has also been reported with HIV infection.[45] Pseudoclubbing of the nail or beaking (increase in longitudinal curvature of the nail with loss of nail plate material) can be seen in scleroderma.[46]

Pincer Nail

Pincer nail clinically is transverse overcurvature of the nail and has been associated with psoriasis, systemic lupus erythematosus, and β-blocker use (**Fig. 5**)[39]

Pterygium

Pterygium of the nail typically is the presence of a scarred midline band originating from the proximal nail fold in the nail and has been seen in graft-versus-host-disease (**Fig. 6**).[39] Pterygium inversum unguis, where the distal nail bed fuses to the ventral nail plate, can be seen in systemic sclerosis,[39] systemic lupus erythematosus,[39] and dermatomysoitis.[46] Pitting of the nail can also be seen in systemic sclerosis.[46]

Melanonychia

Dark pigmentation of the nail caused by melanin is called "melanonychia."[39,44] Multiple longitudinal bands of melanonychia can be racial or caused by medications.[39] The abnormality has also been reported in Peutz-Jeghers syndrome, AIDS, Laugier-Huntziker syndrome, Addison disease, and pregnancy.[39,44] A single longitudinal band should be biopsied to exclude a nail apparatus melanoma.[39,44]

Leukonychia

Leukonychia is defined as white discoloration of the nail plate caused by abnormal keratinization of the distal nail matrix (**Fig. 7**).[39,44] It can affect the whole nail plate (leukonychia totalis) and be hereditary or be caused by cirrhosis and ulcerative colitis.[39] If it only affects part of the nail (leukonychia partialis) it can be caused by metastatic carcinoma, Hodgkin disease, or nephritis.[39] Leprosy can cause leukonychia totalis

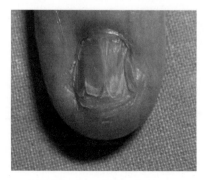

Fig. 5. Pincer nail.

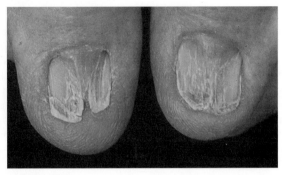

Fig. 6. Pterygium of nail.

or partialis.[39] Kawasaki disease can demonstrate leukonychia partialis, leukonychia striata, and other nail changes of Beau lines, nail loss, and pincer nail deformity.[47] Punctate and striate leukonychia are often caused by nail trauma.[44] Mees lines are transverse white bands of the nail that can be seen in cardiac failure, renal failure, arsenic or thallium ingestion, and Hodgkin disease.[39,48]

Half-and-half Nails

Half-and-half nails are seen in chronic renal failure, with the proximal part being opaque white in color and the distal area of the nail (20%–60%) red.[39] It has also been seen in Crohn disease[49] and HIV patients.[45]

Terry Nails

The proximal nail is opaque white in color with only a small 1- to 2-mm band of reddish brown discoloration at the distal free edge of the nail.[39] Diabetes mellitus, hepatic disorders, and congestive heart failure have been associated.[39,44] In addition, they have been seen with HIV infection[45] and hemodialysis patients.[50]

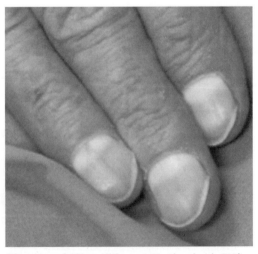

Fig. 7. Leukonychia. (*Courtesy of* Alison Vidmos, MD, Cleveland, OH.)

Muehrcke White Bands

Muehrcke white bands are seen in hypoalbuminemic states, such as nephritic syndrome and liver disease, and are two whites lines parallel to the lunula extending across the nail with an intervening middle pink-red band.[39,50]

Red Lunula

Erythema of the lunula is a nonspecific finding and is seen in diseases of different body systems.[39] It can be observed in cardiac failure, liver cirrhosis, and chronic obstructive pulmonary disease.[50] Blue lunula can be seen in Wilson disease and argyria.[50]

Macronychia

An enlarged nail compared with surrounding digits can be found in acromegaly.[39]

Micronychia

A smaller nail compared with surrounding digits can be found in hyperparathyroidism and acromegaly.[39]

Splinter Hemorrhages

Splinter hemorrhages are caused by leaking of the longitudinally oriented blood vessels on the nail bed and clinically are seen as nonblanchable, dark red or brown or black thin longitudinal lines under the nail (**Fig. 8**).[44,50] Splinter hemorrhages can be seen with bacterial endocarditis,[44,51] antiphospholipid syndrome,[44] liver disease,[50] trichinosis,[50] and scleroderma.[46] Local nail trauma and psoriasis can also cause splinter hemorrhages.[44]

Onycholysis

Onycholysis is defined as division of the distal nail plate from the nail bed (see **Fig. 8**).[39] It can occur in hypothyroidism, with chemotherapy and pellagra.[39] "Plummer's nails" or onycholysis of the fourth and fifth digits are seen in hyperthyroidism.[39,50] Primary systemic amyloidosis can also cause onycholysis, and other nail changes of brittle nails and striation and subungual thickening.[52] Local nail infection or trauma can also cause onycholysis.[44]

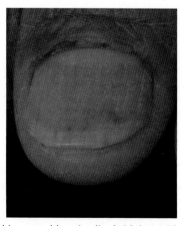

Fig. 8. Mild onycholysis and increased longitudinal ridging with splinter hemorrhages.

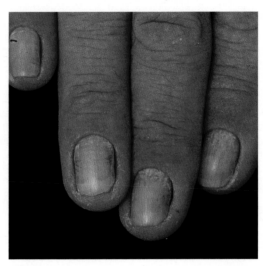

Fig. 9. Yellow nail syndrome.

Beading of the Nail

Beading of the nail can be seen with scleroderma and rheumatoid arthritis and demonstrates discrete tear-drop shaped depressions in the nail plate.[46]

Nail Fold Capillary Changes

Normal nail fold capillaries are small, even, and organized. With scleroderma, the capillaries enlarge, become disorganized and bleed, and later disappear in areas.[46] Similar changes are seen in dermatomyositis and mixed connective tissue disease.[46] In systemic lupus erythematosus, the nail fold capillaries are tortuous and can resemble glomeruli of the kidney.[44,46]

Ragged Cuticles

Ragged torn cuticles are seen in connective tissue diseases, such as scleroderma.[46] Hyperkeratotic cuticles are seen also in dermatomyositis and systemic lupus erythematosus.[44] Hemorrhagic nails can be seen with pemphigus vulgaris.[53]

Yellow Nail Syndrome

Nails are overcurved, thickened, and opaque yellow to yellowish green (**Fig. 9**).[39,44] It has been reported as a paraneoplastic process, but more commonly is a syndrome with features of lymphoedema, respiratory disease, and yellow nails.[39] Respiratory manifestations can be pleural effusions, bronchiectasis, chronic sinusitis, or recurrent pneumonia.[54]

SUMMARY

The hair and nails are rapidly growing structures and as such their cell division can be interrupted by disease states and iatrogenic treatments. Other internal diseases can alter the structure and color of the hair and nails. These alterations in the hair and nails supply important information to the physician regarding the underlying diagnosis.

REFERENCES

1. Kligman AM. Pathologic dynamics of human hair loss. I. Telogen effluvium. Arch Dermatol 1961;83:175–98.
2. Headington JE. Telogen effluvium: new concepts and review. Arch Dermatol 1992;129:356–63.
3. Cotsarelis G, Millar S, Chan EF. Embryology and anatomy of the hair follicle. In: Olsen EA, editor. Disorders of hair growth: diagnosis and treatment. 2nd edition. New York: McGraw-Hill Publishing; 2003. p. 23–48.
4. Paus R, Cotsarelis G. The biology of hair follicles. N Engl J Med 1999;341:491–7.
5. Rook A, Dawber R. Diffuse alopecia: endocrine, metabolic and chemical influences on the follicular cycle. In: Rook A, Dawber R, editors. Diseases of the hair and scalp. Oxford, UK: Blackwell Scientific Publications; 1982. p. 115–45.
6. Goette DU, Odum RB. Alopecia in crash dieters. JAMA 1976;235:2622–3.
7. Bergfeld WF. Telogen effluvium. In: McMichael AJ, Hordinsky MK, editors. Hair and scalp diseases: medical, surgical and cosmetic treatments. New York: Informa Healthcare; 2008. p. 119–35.
8. Apache PG. Eczematous dermatitis of the scalp. In: Zviak C, editor. The science of hair care. New York: Marcel Dekker; 1986. p. 513–21.
9. Fiedler VC, Gray AC. Diffuse alopecia: telogen hair loss. In: Olsen EA, editor. Disorders of hair growth: diagnosis and treatment. 2nd edition. USA: McGraw-Hill Publishing; 2003. p. 303–20.
10. Sperling LC. Hair and systemic disease. Dermatol Clin 2001;19(4):711–26.
11. Freinkel R, Freinkel N. Hair growth and alopecia in hypothyroidism. Arch Dermatol 1972;106(3):349–52.
12. Saito R, Hori Y, Kuribayashi T. Alopecia in hypothyroidism. In: Kobori T, Montagna W, editors. Biology of diseases of the hair. Tokyo: University of Tokyo Press; 1976. p. 279–85.
13. Johnson AA, Latham MC, Roe DA. An evaluation of the use of changes in hair root morphology in the assessment of protein-caloric malnutrition. Am J Clin Nutr 1976;29:502–11.
14. Rushton DH, Ramsey ID. The importance of adequate serum ferritin levels during oral cyproterone acetate and ethinyl oestradiol treatment of diffuse androgen deoendent alopecia in women. Clin Endocrinol 1992;36:421–7.
15. Trost LB, Bergfeld WF, Calogeras E. The diagnosis and treatment of iron deficiency and its potential relationship to hair loss. J Am Acad Dermatol 2006;54:824–44.
16. Vegesna V, O'Kelly J, Uskokovic M, et al. Vitamin D3 analogs stimulate hair growth in nude mice. Endocrinology 2002;143(11):4389–96.
17. Whiting DA. Chronic telogen effluvium. Dermatol Clin 1996;14:723–73.
18. Whiting DA. Chronic telogen effluvium: increased scalp hair shedding in middle-aged women. J Am Acad Dermatol 1996;35(6):899–906.
19. Tosti A, Pazzaglia M. Drug reactions affecting hair: diagnosis. Dermatol Clin 2007;25:223–31.
20. Ross EK, Shapiro J. Management of hair loss. Dermatol Clin 2005;23:227–43.
21. Sinclair R, Grossman KL, Kvedar JC. Anagen hair loss. In: Olsen EA, editor. Disorders of hair growth: diagnosis and treatment. 3rd edition. New York: McGraw-Hill Publishing; 2003. p. 123–75.
22. Madani S, Shapiro J. Alopecia areata update. J Am Acad Dermatol 2000;42:549–66.
23. Olsen EA, Messenger AG, Shapiro J, et al. Evaluation and treatment of male and female pattern hair loss. J Am Acad Dermatol 2005;52:301–11.

24. Hamilton JB. Male hormone stimulation is prerequisite and an incitant in common baldness. Am J Anat 1942;71:451–80.

25. Futterweit MD, Dunaif A, Yeh H-C, et al. The prevalence of hyperandrogenism in 109 consecutive female patients with diffuse alopecia. J Am Acad Dermatol 1988;19:831–6.

26. Sperling LC, Lupton GP. Histopathology of non-scarring alopecia. J Cutan Pathol 1995;22(2):97–114.

27. Lesko SM, Rosenberg L, Shapiro S. A case-control study of baldness in relation to myocardial infarction in men. JAMA 1993;269:9987–10003.

28. Carey AH, Chan KL, Short F, et al. Evidence for a single gene effect causing polycystic ovaries and male pattern baldness. Clin Endocrinol 1993;38:653–8.

29. Mofid A, Seyyed Alinaghi SA, Zandieh S, et al. Hirsutism. Int J Clin Pract 2008; 62(3):433–43 [Epub 2007 Dec 11].

30. Rosenfield RL. Clinical practice: hirsutism. N Engl J Med 2005;353(24):2578–88.

31. Azziz R, Waggoner WT, Ochoa T, et al. Idiopathic hirsutism: an uncommon cause of hirsutism in Alabama. Fertil Steril 1998;70(2):274–8.

32. The Rotterdam ESHRE/ASRM-Sponsored PCOS Consensus Workshop Group. Revised 2003 consensus on diagnostic criteria and long-term health risks related to polycystic ovary syndrome (PCOS). Hum Reprod 2004;19(1):41–7.

33. Azziz R, Woods KS, Reyna R, et al. The prevalence and features of the polycystic ovary syndrome in an unselected population. J Clin Endocrinol Metab 2004;89(6): 2745–9.

34. Derman RJ. Androgen excess in women. Int J Fertil Menopausal Stud 1996;41(2): 172–6.

35. Martin KA, Chang RJ, Ehrmann DA, et al. Evaluation and treatment of hirsutism in premenopausal women: an Endocrine Society Clinical Practice Guideline. J Clin Endocrinol Metab 2008;93(4):1105–20.

36. Practice Committee of the American Society for Reproductive Medicine. The evaluation and treatment of androgen excess. Fertil Steril 2006;86(4 Suppl):S241–7.

37. Olsen EA. Hypertrichosis. In: Olsen EA, editor. Disorders of hair growth: diagnosis and treatment. 3rd edition. New York: McGraw-Hill Publishing; 2003. p. 123–75.

38. Whiting DA. Hair shaft defects. In: Olsen EA, editor. Disorders of hair growth: diagnosis and treatment. 3rd edition. New York: McGraw-Hill Publishing; 2003. p. 123–75.

39. Ramos-e-Silva M, Azevedo-e-Silva MC, Carneiro SC. Hair, nail and pigment changes in major systemic disease. Clin Dermatol 2008;26:296–305.

40. Harries MJ, Sinclair RD, MacDonald-Hull S, et al. Management of primary cicatricial alopecias: options for treatment. Br J Dermatol 2008;159(1):1–22.

41. Headington JT. Cicatricial alopecia. Dermatol Clin 1996;14(4):773–82.

42. Selva D, Chen CS, James CL, et al. Discoid lupus erythematosus presenting as madarosis. Am J Ophthalmol 2003;136(3):545–6.

43. Somani N, Bergfeld WF. Classification and histopathologic findings of the cicatricial alopecias. Dermatol Ther 2008;21(4):221–37.

44. Tosti A, Piraccini BM. Biology of the nails and nail disorders. In: Wolff K, Goldsmith LA, Katz SI, et al, editors. Fitzpatrick's dermatology in general medicine. 7th edition. New York: McGraw Hill Companies Inc; 2008. p. 778–94.

45. Cribier B, Mena ML, Rey D, et al. Nail changes in patients infected with human immunodeficiency virus: a prospective controlled study. Arch Dermatol 1998; 134:1216–20.

46. Sherber NS, Wigley FM, Scher RK. Autoimmune disorders: nail signs and therapeutic approaches. Dermatol Ther 2007;20:17–30.

47. Berard R, Scuccimarri R, Chedeville G. Leukonychia striata in Kawasaki disease: case report. J Pediatr 2008;152(6):889.
48. Chauchan S, D'Cruz S, Singh R, et al. Mee's lines:case report. Lancet 2008; 372(9647):1410.
49. Zagoni T, Sipos F, Tarjan Z, et al. The half-and-half nail: a new sign of Crohn's disease? Report of four cases. Dis Colon Rectum 2006;49:1071–3.
50. Gregariou S, Argyriou G, Larios G, et al. Nail disorders and systemic disease: what the nails tell us. J Fam Pract 2008;57(8):509–14.
51. Ferris LK, English JC III. The skin in infective endocarditis, sepsis, septic shock, and disseminated intravascular coagulation. In: Wolff K, Goldsmith LA, Katz SI, et al, editors. Fitzpatrick's dermatology in general medicine. 7th edition. New York: McGraw Hill Companies Inc; 2008. p. 1744–9.
52. Prat C, Moreno A, Vinas M, et al. Nail dystrophy in primary systemic amyloidosis [letter]. J Eur Acad Dermatol Venereol 2008;22(1):107–9.
53. Reich A, Wisnicka B, Szepietowski JC. Haemorrhagic nails in pemphigus vulgaris [letter]. Acta Derm Venereol 2008;88(5):542.
54. Maldonado F, Tazelaar HD, Wang CW, et al. Yellow nail syndrome: analysis of 41 patients. Chest 2008;134(2):375–81.

Allergic Skin Disease: Major Highlights and Recent Advances

Kim M. Nichols, MD[a], Fran E. Cook-Bolden, MD[a,b],*

KEYWORDS

- Atopic dermatitis • Urticaria • Allergic contact dermatitis
- Allergic skin diseases • Atopy • Eczema

ATOPIC DERMATITIS

Atopic dermatitis (AD) is a chronic inflammatory pruritic disease that affects 2% to 5% of the general population, including 10% to 20% of children and approximately 1% to 3% of adults.[1] The prevalence of AD has increased steadily since World War II, and seems to be rising in most industrialized countries.[2] More than 60% to 80% of AD cases present before the first year of life, and in 95% of cases, occurs before age 5 years.[3] A small proportion of patients do not present with AD until adulthood. AD has no racial predilection, although African Americans and Asian-Americans visit the doctor more frequently for symptoms.[4] Although maternal history of atopy is one of the strongest predictors of AD, environmental factors clearly play a significant role in the pathogenesis of the disease. More severe disease is seen in urban areas and in children who have early age of onset and an associated respiratory allergy.[5] It is more prevalent in patients from an advantaged socioeconomic class. Furthermore, although it is seen in all countries, it has a higher incidence in developed nations and in fact, its frequency is increased in patients who immigrate to developed countries from underdeveloped countries.[6]

Why atopic dermatitis is more prevalent in developed areas is not completely understood. However, many believe that it is explained by the "hygiene hypothesis," which was first proposed by David Strachan[7] in 1989. He suggested that early childhood infections allow children to develop the necessary immune protection against atopic diseases, such as eczema, asthma, food allergies, and allergic rhinitis. Consequently, children in developed countries, especially those in urban areas, who grow up without significant exposure to microbes are at higher risk for these conditions.[8] Additionally, recent studies have shown a link between exposure to antibiotics in the first year of life

[a] Skin Specialty Group, 150 East 58th Street, 3rd Floor Annex, New York, NY 10155, USA
[b] Department of Dermatology, College of Physicians and Surgeons of Columbia University, 630 West 168th Street, P&S 3-401, New York, NY 10032, USA
* Corresponding author. Skin Specialty Group, 150 East 58th Street, 3rd Floor Annex, New York, NY 10155.
E-mail address: admin.skinspecialtygroup@gmail.com (F.E. Cook-Bolden).

Med Clin N Am 93 (2009) 1211–1224
doi:10.1016/j.mcna.2009.08.004
0025-7125/09/$ – see front matter © 2009 Elsevier Inc. All rights reserved.

and subsequent development of atopic dermatitis. At a recent meeting of the European Society for Dermatological Research, Dr Jochen Schmitt[9] of Germany reported that in a prospective population-based study involving 370 children in Saxony, Germany, exposure to antibiotics in the first year of life was associated with a 66% increased likelihood of developing AD in the second year. These findings were dose-related, with children prescribed one course of antibiotics in their first year having a 1.5-fold increased risk for developing AD, and those prescribed two or more courses having a 2.1-fold increased risk. In his report, Dr Schmitt noted that his results were in line with a previous larger study whose report in 2000 showed that exposure to antibiotics in the first year of life was associated with a 30% increased risk for developing AD by 7 to 8 years of age.[9] Finally, although not all studies support the hygiene hypothesis,[7] cumulative evidence now shows that environmental factors, such as early infections, early allergen exposure, outdoor and indoor pollution, and diet, may play a vital role in atopic disease expression.[10]

Infantile AD is characterized by generalized xerosis and erythematous scaly exudative plaques affecting the cheeks, forehead, scalp, and extensor extremities. Often the diaper area is spared. As the disease progresses into childhood, lesions tend to migrate to the flexure areas, particularly the antecubital and popliteal fossae, and the creases of the buttocks and thighs. At this point, lichenification and excoriations begin to appear, secondary to chronic scratching and rubbing of the skin. In addition, telltale signs of AD may manifest, such as pityriasis alba of the face and Dennie-Morgan lines (ie, increased hyperpigmentation and wrinkles below the eyes). Among infants and children who have moderate to severe AD, 40% will also develop food allergies, with cow's milk, eggs, peanuts, and soy the most common offenders.[11] By adulthood, 40% to 80% of patients who have AD will experience either a decrease or complete resolution of their disease. However, despite this regression, many adults who have AD exhibit the sequelae of a history of eczema, including chronic lichenification, hyperpigmented patches resulting from previous excoriations, and the "dirty neck" sign: a brown macular ring around the neck that represents a localized deposition of amyloid. Additionally, up to 70% of adults who have a history of AD will also have a respiratory allergy.[12]

The diagnosis of AD is based on a constellation of signs and symptoms, not a specific test or laboratory marker. In 2003, Eichenfield and colleagues[13] published a suggested set of diagnostic criteria for AD that they presented at an American Academy of Dermatology consensus conference on pediatric AD. Essential features for diagnosis included pruritus and eczematous changes that were acute, subacute, and chronic. In addition, important features seen in most cases of AD were early age of onset, atopy, and xerosis. Furthermore, associated but nonspecific features included keratosis pilaris, lichenification, and periorbital changes. Finally, the consensus board indicated that a firm diagnosis of AD should be made only if other similar conditions, such as seborrheic dermatitis, scabies, psoriasis, and allergic contact dermatitis, have been thoroughly excluded.

The exact cause of atopic dermatitis is still poorly understood. Recent research has shown that AD involves a complicated interplay between genetic predisposition, immune responses, epithelial barrier dysfunction, infectious agents, and environmental factors. The role of genetics in AD has long been of interest to researchers. Patients who have AD have a strong family history of AD and other atopic diseases. In a study of 372 AD patients, a positive family history of atopy was present in 73% of cases.[14] In addition, studies have detected a high concordance in monozygotic twin pairs.[15] In light of these clinical findings, researchers have been prompted to investigate the specific genes involved in atopy and in AD, in particular. Genomic scans have identified several susceptibility genes, including loci on chromosomes 5q31–33, 3q21, 1q21, 16q, 17q25, and 20p, which code for interleukin (IL)-4 and other T helper 2 (Th2) cell cytokines involved in IgE synthesis.[16] Other candidate genes discovered include one on chromosome 11q13, which codes for the high-affinity IgE receptor (FcεRI) found in AD lesional skin.[17]

Researchers have also discovered *SPINK5* mutations in two families who have a strong history of AD. *SPINK5* mutations are most closely related to Netherton syndrome, a genodermatosis that presents with an atopic diathesis, trichorrhexis invaginata, and ichthyosis linearis circumflexa.[18]

In terms of the immune abnormalities seen in AD, it has long been accepted that skin lesions in AD result from an imbalance between Th2 and Th1 lymphocytes. Acute AD lesions exhibit reduced expression of IL-12 and increased production of IL-10, which increases Th2 activity and suppresses Th1 activity.[2] This mechanism results in cytokine production of IL-4, -5, -12, and -13, which causes an increase in IgE and a decrease in interferon (IFN)-γ levels. Consequently, patients who have acute AD have a cutaneous immunodeficiency that makes them more susceptible to infection, such as herpes simplex virus and molluscum. In addition, epidermal Langerhans cells in atopic skin have several high-affinity IgE receptors that, when triggered, further promote the IgE-mediated hypersensitivity and inflammatory responses seen in AD.

This IgE reactivity has led many to describe AD as an atopic disease, with *atopy* defined as "a form of allergy in which there is a genetic predisposition to develop hypersensitivity reactions (eg, hay fever, allergic asthma, or atopic eczema) in response to allergens."[19] However, the term *atopic* has been the source of much controversy relating to the nomenclature of AD. As Simpson and Hanifin[2] mention in a recent article, although 80% of adults who have AD exhibit high serum IgE levels, approximately 10% to 20% have normal IgE levels. These investigators question whether AD should be considered strictly a disease of allergic etiology. They contend that rather than being caused by allergies, AD should be viewed as skin disease that predisposes to allergies. In fact, they propose a new comprehensive definition of atopy that would account for the varying levels of IgE reactivity seen in AD: "a genetically predisposed diathesis manifesting as exaggerated responses (eg, bronchoconstriction, IgE production, vasodilatation, pruritus) to a variety of environmental stimuli (irritants, allergens, and microbes)."[2]

With the role of atopy in atopic dermatitis under debate, many researchers have been prompted to explore the roles of multiple other factors in the pathogenesis of the disease. Of particular interest has been the epithelial barrier dysfunction exhibited in AD. Experts have long accepted that AD skin is characterized by severe xerosis and increased transepidermal water loss, even in nonlesional skin.[20] Many studies have shown that this water loss may be caused by a deficiency of ceramide in AD skin. Ceramide is a crucial structural component of sphingolipids and functions to retain water in the skin. In a recent study, investigators found that sphingomyelin deacylase activity was significantly increased in the epidermis of patients who had AD and contact dermatitis compared with controls. This increased sphingomyelin deacylase expression is believed to lead to a metabolism of ceramide and subsequent ceramide deficiency. Consequently, the stratum corneum in AD skin loses much of its water-binding capacity.[21]

The stratum corneum in AD is also affected by mutations in the genes that encode filaggrin, the main protein component of keratohyalin granules. Filaggrin is essential to the formation of the cornified envelope, which is the basis of normal barrier function in the skin. Filaggrin mutations are known to occur in ichthyosis vulgaris. However, multiple studies have also recently discovered loss-of-function null mutations in atopic dermatitis.[22] Filaggrin mutations have been associated with early-onset eczema, allergy sensitization, and eczema-associated asthma. And in one study, Howell and colleagues[23] found that many patients who had AD exhibited low filaggrin expression even if they did not have full loss-of-function mutations.

These findings of filaggrin dysfunction, coupled with evidence of ceramide deficiency in AD skin, have led many investigators to conclude that epidermal barrier disruption is the primary cause of AD; that, in fact, the breakdown of the skin barrier is what drives allergic sensitization and skin inflammation in AD, not the converse, which has been the conventional belief. These alterations in the stratum corneum allow penetration of irritants and allergens, which spark the inflammatory cascade, hypersensitivity, and skin damage seen in AD.[17] Consequently, studies have now focused on the development of new modalities aimed at repairing the epidermal barrier dysfunction, which lies at the root of AD pathophysiology.

Although many new and exciting therapies for AD are being developed, educating patients and their families begins with a discussion of prevention. Because a maternal history of atopy increases the risk for having an atopic child, many studies have looked at whether maternal allergen avoidance in pregnancy can prevent the development of AD in children. A Cochrane systematic review of these studies concluded that maternal dietary changes and allergy avoidance in pregnancy did not seem to confer a protective effect against AD.[24] Breastfeeding has also been identified as having the potential to reduce allergen exposure in newborns and prevent AD. However, after reviewing multiple studies, the American Association of Dermatology Guidelines Task Force in 2004 reported that no conclusive evidence showed that breastfeeding prevented AD.[25]

More hopeful results have emerged from recent research into the use of probiotics in utero and in newborns. In line with the hygiene hypothesis, investigators have theorized that probiotics may reverse the permeability of the gut epithelium to allergic antigens, thus providing a protective effect against atopic disease. And in fact, a 4-year follow-up study by Kalliomaki and colleagues[26] found that when pregnant women who had atopic histories and their newborns were given probiotics (in the form of *Lactobacillus acidophilus*), the incidence of AD in the children was significantly reduced (23% in the test group compared with 46% in the control).

In a 2008 meta-analysis of six prevention and four treatment double-blind, randomized, controlled trials of probiotics and pediatric AD, the authors reported a significant risk reduction (by as much as 61%) associated with the use of prenatal or postnatal probiotics for the primary prevention of pediatric AD among 1581 participants. However, because only a marginal effect was seen in the treatment group, the researchers concluded that although prenatal probiotics may play a role in AD prevention, they do not seem to be effective in the treatment of pediatric AD.[27]

As the possibilities of primary prevention of AD continue to be explored, currently patients must focus on optimal disease management, which begins with proper skin hydration. Most patients are advised that ideally, a petroleum-based moisturizer should be applied to the entire body within 3 minutes of bathing at least once, but preferably twice, a day. During flares, most patients are also treated with a topical corticosteroids or topical calcineurin-inhibitors for short periods. To prevent corticosteroid-induced complications, topical corticosteroids are often used on an "on/off" rotation: twice a day for 2 weeks "on" and 2 weeks "off." Many dermatologists agree that to get rapid control of a flare, it is better to use a short 1- to 2-week course of a mid-potency topical corticosteroid rather than a long course of suboptimal low-potency topical corticosteroids. However, once remission is achieved, maintenance therapy involves the generous use of topical emollients, topical calcineurin inhibitors, and perhaps once-weekly or "weekend" use of topical corticosteroids. When relapse occurs, patients return to twice-daily applications of higher-potency topical corticosteroids for short periods.

Although petroleum-based moisturizers are most often recommended by providers, patient compliance is often low because of the inelegant nature of these products. Therefore, several emollient products recently have entered the market that are not only more cosmetically acceptable but also specifically engineered to improve the skin barrier dysfunction in AD. One of the first lines of products to emerge has been ceramide-based moisturizers, designed to replace the ceramides deficient in the stratum corneum of AD skin. Among the lines are CeraVe (Coria Laboratories, Ltd, Aliso Viejo, California), Proderm (Quinnova Pharmaceuticals, Inc, Newtown, Pennsylvania), and TriCeram (Osmotics Pharmaceutical Corp, Wilmington, North Carolina).[28]

An open-label study published in 2002 showed dramatic improvements in clinical activity, permeability barrier function, and stratum corneum integrity when the over-the-counter version of this technology (TriCeram) was substituted for standard moisturizers in children who had severe recalcitrant AD.[29] In 2008, a new ceramide-based FDA-approved product entered the market called EpiCeram (Ceragenix Pharmaceuticals, Inc, Denver, Colorado). EpiCeram is a combination of ceramides, cholesterols, and fatty acids. A multicenter, randomized study compared 4 weeks of twice-daily EpiCeram with fluticasone propionate in children who had moderate to severe atopic dermatitis. They found that, although at day 14 subjects in the fluticasone group had significantly better Scoring Atopic Dermatitis (SCORAD) scores compared with the EpiCeram group, by day 28 no significant differences were seen in the SCORAD scores between the groups. The manufacturers claim that although it is slow to start working, EpiCeram may decrease the need for topical corticosteroids and may ultimately, through its restoration of the skin lipid barrier, decrease the number and severity of flares.[30,31]

Other barrier products recently introduced include MimyX (Stiefel Laboratories, Inc, Coral Gables, Florida) and Atopiclair (Graceway Pharmaceuticals, LLC, Bristol, Tennessee). Both products are 510(k) medical devices that have been cleared for marketing by the FDA. Mimyx is a palmitamide monoethanolamine (PEA)–containing nonsteroidal and topical calcineurin inhibitor-free cream designed to replace PEA deficient in atopic skin. In a study of 2500 subjects who had AD, researchers found that adding Mimyx to the subjects' daily regimens significantly improved symptoms. In addition, it increased the time between flares compared with emollients alone, improved patients' sleep quality, and was steroid-sparing.[32] Atopiclair, or MAS063, is a nonsteroidal topical cream that contains glycyrrhetinic acid, hyaluronic acid, grape leaf extract, telmesteine, and Shea butter.

In a multicenter, randomized vehicle-controlled study, researchers compared MAS063 to vehicle alone in the treatment of 106 infants and children who had mild to moderate atopic dermatitis. Pruritus; Eczema Area and Severity Index (EASI) scores; subject and caregiver assessment of global response; onset and duration of itch relief; and need for rescue medication were all significantly improved in the treatment group compared with the vehicle group.[33] The role of topical barrier products in the management of AD is still to be fully ascertained.

Although these preliminary studies show that these products may be helpful as adjuvant therapy in AD, better studies must be performed to support these initial reports.

Like the cornified envelope, the antimicrobial barrier is also compromised in patients who have AD. Although failure of both permeability and antimicrobial function is well recognized in patients who have AD, the fact that these two functions are interdependent has only recently become clear. As Elias and colleagues[34] mention in a recent review article, "… the failure of the permeability barrier in itself favors secondary infection, and conversely, pathogen colonization/infection further aggravates the permeability barrier abnormality."

Colonization by *Staphylococcus aureus* is almost universal in AD, and is seen in 90% of patients. Secondary infections are common, such as impetiginization, widespread folliculitis, or, less frequently, cutaneous abscesses or cellulitis. Furthermore, colonization by superantigen-producing *S aureus* strains further exacerbates disease in patients who have severe AD through generalized augmentation of IgE production and through development of specific IgE directed toward staphylococcal exotoxins.[2] Patients who have AD are also more susceptible to widespread cutaneous viral infections, including molluscum contagiosum, herpes simplex (Kaposi's varicelliform eruption), and vaccinia, and exhibit increased incidence of widespread tinea corporis and *Malassezia* spp infections.[35]

Although oral antibiotics have long been a mainstay in the treatment of severe AD flares, recent studies have evaluated the efficacy of topical antiseptics in the prevention and treatment of the disease. Topical antiseptics, such as triclosan and chlorhexidine, which have a low sensitizing potential and low resistance rate compared with topical antibiotics, have been studied as an adjunctive therapy to topical corticosteroids.[35] In one randomized, double-blind, controlled trial, investigators assessed the safety and efficacy of a novel triclosan-incorporated emollient cream to its vehicle. They found the emollient cream was a safe adjunctive treatment in AD but did not significantly improve the outcomes compared with the vehicle group.[36] In another study, fusidic acid proved to be very effective against *S aureus* infections in AD, but was most effective when used for treatment periods longer than 2 weeks.[35]

In addition to these new topical modalities for AD, several novel systemic treatments are being studied. These include the use of low-dose anti-IgE therapy. The IgE-blocking antibody omalizumab (Xolair, Novartis Pharmaceuticals, Basel, Switzerland) is an FDA-approved drug used to treat patients 12 years and older who have moderate to severe persistent asthma.

Omalizumab is a recombinant humanized monoclonal antibody that blocks IgE's high-affinity Fc receptor.[32] Omalizumab stops free-serum IgE from attaching to mast cells and other immune cells and prevents IgE-mediated inflammatory changes.[37] In one study, Belloni and colleagues[38] found that omalizumab reduced the SCORAD in 6 of 11 patients. In another case study of three children who had severe recalcitrant AD with extremely high IgE levels (1900–6120 IU/mL), Lane and colleagues[39] saw a significant improvement in the patients' disease. These investigators concluded that omalizumab may be a safe and effective therapeutic option in patients who have severe AD, especially those who have high IgE levels.

Although treatment of AD with omalizumab may be considered cutting-edge by some researchers, others are pushing the boundaries even further. At an atopic dermatitis symposium at the American Academy of Dermatology 2008 summer meeting, Dr Albert Yan[40] from Chicago described three innovative therapies being researched in AD. The first was whole-body cryotherapy, which has been used since the 1970s to treat rheumatic pain. Finnish researchers theorized that because whole-body cryotherapy slows down acetylcholine synthesis in peripheral nerves and has antioxidative properties, it may be improve pruritus in AD. In a small study with 18 adults, they found that it reduced SCORAD scores by 20%.[41]

The second experimental treatment discussed by Dr Yan was vitamin D supplementation. In a pilot study examining the effect of 1000 IU of oral ergocalciferol (vitamin D) supplementation in a group of children who had mild to severe AD, Sidbury[42] showed that vitamin D supplementation moderately improved wintertime onset or exacerbation. Investigators explained these findings as being caused partly by the ability of vitamin D to induce expression of antimicrobial peptides that help prevent skin infection associated with AD exacerbations.

The third novel therapy was rosiglitazone (Avandia, GlaxoSmithKline, Brentford, Middlesex, United Kingdom). Rosiglitazone, which is approved for use in type II diabetes, is believed to have anti-inflammatory properties that might be therapeutic in AD. However, the results in three past studies have not been promising; only in one recent study was rosiglitazone associated with a mild decrease in symptoms in patients who had severe AD who had been recalcitrant to first- and second-line therapies. And for most subjects, this effect took at least 2 to 3 months to manifest.[40]

URTICARIA

Unlike atopic dermatitis, urticaria is believed to have a more clear-cut allergic or immune-mediated pathogenesis. Urticaria affects an estimated 15% to 20% of people at some point in their lives. It also accounts for approximately 50% of all emergency department visits related to a skin disorder. More than 80% of cases of new-onset urticaria resolve in 2 weeks and greater than 95% of new-onset cases resolve within 3 months. Urticarial episodes are characterized by the onset of wheals (hives) and pruritus. The individual lesions are erythematous, evanescent papules, and plaques that may show central clearing and an advancing migratory border. By definition, the lesions last less than 24 hours and heal without scarring. When individual lesions last more than 36 to 48 hours and leave postinflammatory hyperpigmentation or palpable purpura, the diagnosis of urticarial vasculitis is more likely. Acute urticaria is defined as having symptomatic episodes lasting up to 6 weeks. When symptoms last longer than 6 weeks, the disorder is termed *chronic urticaria*.[43–45]

In 50% of cases of urticaria, a specific cause is identified. The most common cause of acute urticaria is respiratory infection, believed to account for 39% of cases. Other causes include medications (eg, nonsteroidal anti-inflammatory drugs, antibiotics, opiates, angiotensin converting enzyme inhibitors); foods (eg, nuts, shellfish, strawberries); parasitic infections; arthropod bites; and intravenous radiocontrast media. Many types of physical urticaria exist (which is usually chronic), including dermatographic, cholinergic, cold, and delayed-pressure urticaria. Urticaria can also be a symptom of an autoimmune systemic disease, such as hypo- or hyperthyroidism. Rarely, urticaria is paraneoplastic or part of a syndrome, such as Schnitzler or Muckle-Wells syndrome.[45,46] However, in half of all cases of urticaria, a definitive cause cannot be found, especially in chronic urticaria, in which unexplained cases are termed *chronic idiopathic urticaria* (CIU).

The mast cell is the central mediator in the pathogenesis of urticaria. In acute allergic urticaria, mast cells and basophils are triggered by the crosslinking of IgE (bound to the mast cell surface at the FcεRI receptor) and a specific antigen. Mast cell degranulation ensues and histamine, leukotriene C4, prostaglandin D2, and other chemotactic medicators are released, leading to wheal formation, vasodilation, and erythema. In addition, eosinophils and neutrophils are recruited, which further promote wheal formation.

In chronic urticaria, the pathogenesis is more complex. Recent research has shown that CIU may be more of an autoimmune rather than allergic phenomena. Approximately one third of patients who have chronic urticaria have antithyroid (antithyroglobulin or antimicrosomal) antibodies, and these antibodies have now been shown to have pathogenic significance.[47] In a recent review of multiple studies on this subject, investigators found that 35% to 40% of the cases were caused by an IgG antibody recognizing a portion of the cell-surface high-affinity IgE receptor, and an additional 5% to 10% were caused by IgG antibody binding to IgE itself.[48] This autoimmune reaction is believed to cause chronic stimulation and degranulation by mast cells, thus explaining cases of CIU in which a specific allergen is undetectable.

Because of the high prevalence of idiopathic urticaria, new cases of urticaria (especially chronic cases) are often evaluated with an exhaustive workup. This workup often includes a physical examination, including a test for dermatographism; a complete blood cell count to detect abnormalities associated with malignancy and infection; an eosinophil count, which can be linked to parasite infection if elevated; erythrocyte sedimentation rate and antinuclear antibodies, which may be elevated in people who have urticarial vasculitis; stool ova and parasites examination; a test of the serum for cryoglobulin, which can be elevated in some forms of cold-induced urticaria; a test for hepatitis B and C virus, which can be associated with cryoglobulinemia; food allergy tests; tests for *Helicobacter pylori*, which has been linked to urticaria in a few studies; complement studies, which can rule out hereditary angioedema; thyroid function tests, including antithyroid microsomal and peroxidase antibody titers; and a skin biopsy if urticarial vasculitis is suspected.[49–51]

However, despite this thorough and often expensive workup, multiple studies have reported that this nondirected testing often has little usefulness in determining the cause of idiopathic urticaria. In a recent review article, Dibbern[46] refers to a large meta-analysis concluding that this comprehensive testing was entirely futile, showing that screening laboratory testing showed only 1.6% occult disease in patients who had CIU.[52] Nondirected food allergy panels seem to be especially fruitless. Food allergies are often the first suspects in cases of acute urticaria, and therefore the allergy-causing foods are usually quickly identified and eliminated from the diet. However, by the time urticaria becomes chronic, food allergies are rarely found to be the culprit. Multiple large studies have shown food allergies to account for less than 5% of CIU cases.[53,54]

Dibbern[46] recommends that in cases of apparent idiopathic urticaria in otherwise healthy patients, rather than continue with more invasive testing, clinicians should simply begin symptomatic treatment for 6 to 12 weeks. He contends that further diagnostic studies should be performed only if symptoms persist after 12 weeks despite treatment. This further testing may include an autologous serum skin test (ASST), which tests for the presence of a positive functional anti-FcεRI autoimmune antibody. The ASST is an intradermal skin test using a centrifuged sample of patients' own serum. It has a sensitivity of approximately 70% and specificity of 80% for autoimmune urticaria.[55,56] With the use of plasma versus serum in the ASST, the positive test rate can be increased from 55% to 86% in patients who have chronic urticaria. However, for unknown reasons the test can remain positive even after resolution of the urticarial symptoms.[57]

Although advances continue in the diagnostic field, little can be reported in the treatment for urticaria. Of course, if a contributing factor can be determined, avoidance of that trigger is paramount. However, often a cause either cannot be identified or cannot be avoided completely (eg, cold or pressure). Therefore, for most patients, antihistamines remain the mainstay of treatment. H1-receptor antihistamines are the most commonly used agents in treating urticaria. Usually therapy begins with the use of low-sedating second-generation H1-antihistamines (eg, loratadine, fexofenadine). If symptomatic relief is not achieved, most providers will add first-generation sedating H1 blockers (eg, hydroxyzine, diphenhydramine), which have a more potent antihistamine effect. However, although controversial, some researchers and clinicians advocate that before adding a sedating H1 blocker to a patient's therapy, higher doses (double or triple the recommended doses) of the low-sedating H1 blockers should be tried first.[58,59]

Whether using first-, second-generation H1 blockers or both, many studies have concluded that taking H1 antihistamines regularly, rather than as-needed, is the best way to prevent symptoms.[60] In more severe and refractory cases, doxepin, which has both anti-H1 and anti-H2 properties, is also sometimes used; however, it is contraindicated in patients who have glaucoma and must be used with caution in elderly patients and in those who have heart disease.

For patients who experience a poor response to antihistamines, several anti-inflammatories and immunosuppressives have been used with varying degrees of success. These include antileukotrienes; tricyclic antidepressants; COX-2 inhibitors; oral adrenergics; steroids; dapsone and colchicine; cyclosporine; and even omalizumab, the humanized monoclonal anti-IgE used as an experimental treatment for atopic dermatitis.[46]

ALLERGIC CONTACT DERMATITIS

Allergic contact dermatitis (ACD) is inflammation of the skin caused by contact with a specific allergen to which a patient has developed allergic sensitization. It should be distinguished from irritant contact dermatitis, which is skin inflammation resulting from contact with a chemical that causes direct keratinocyte damage.[61] ACD is seen in patients who are genetically predisposed and have been previously sensitized to the allergen in question; irritant contact dermatitis, however, can happen to anyone, especially after repeated exposure. The prevalence of contact dermatitis, both allergic and irritant, has been estimated at 13.6 cases per 1000 population. Contact dermatitis is the most common occupational disease in the United States. It accounts for 90% of all skin disorders acquired in the workplace and is estimated to cost $250 million per year in work-related lost productivity, medical care, and disability payments.[62]

ACD is caused by a delayed-type hypersensitivity reaction to a chemical. More than 3000 environmental chemicals have been identified as causing ACD.[63] On first encounter with a chemical or contact allergen responsible for ACD, haptens from these allergens bind to proteins found on epidermal Langerhans cells, beginning the afferent phase of sensitization. Subsequently, these Langerhans cells interact with Th1 cells in the lymph nodes and prompt the release of memory Th1 cells that are now primed for a second exposure to the allergen.[63] This process of initial sensitization takes approximately 10 to 14 days.[64] However, once the allergen is encountered again, the response is much quicker. On subsequent exposure, cloned memory Th1 cells release a multitude of inflammatory cytokines, which lead to the spongiosis and dermal edema characteristic of ACD. This efferent phase typically takes between 12 to 48 hours.[65]

Lesions of ACD will vary depending on the stage of the disease. In general, during the acute phase, lesions are marked by edema, erythema, and vesicle formation. As the vesicles rupture, oozing ensues and papules and plaques appear. In the chronic stage, scaling, lichenification, and excoriations predominate.[64] In addition, patients may show evidence of secondary bacterial infection. The initial site of the dermatitis often provides the best clue regarding the allergic origin. Because they are most often exposed, the face and hands are the most common body parts presenting with ACD.[62] On the face, the forehead and ears are commonly affected by hair dyes and shampoos; the ears are susceptible to metals from earrings and topical otic preparations; eyelids are particularly affected by airborne allergens and nail polish; the cheeks and lips are prone to react to facial cosmetics.

Neck dermatitis is often caused by airborne allergens, cosmetics, fragrances, or metals from jewelry. More than half of all cases of ACD involve the hands, especially in the workplace. Common culprits include foods, cleansing products, occupational chemicals, latex gloves, and metal from jewelry. Although individuals who have atopic dermatitis are prone to having hand dermatitis, it is usually an irritant rather than an allergic variety. And for unknown reasons, atopic patients have a decreased risk for having ACD, in general.[64]

In addition to the face and hands, the lower legs are prone to ACD, especially in patients who have preexisting stasis dermatitis. The chronic inflammation of the skin in stasis dermatitis increases the risk for ACD from topical medications and lotions, which are often applied under occlusion. Other areas affected by ACD include the oral mucosa, which may present with contact stomatitis from dental metals; the perianal area, which may react to sensitizing medications such as benzocaine; and the axillary area from deodorants and formaldehydes, detergents, and dyes in clothing.[62]

In cases of recurrent or chronic contact dermatitis, the epicutaneous patch test is required to identify possible allergens. Most dermatologists perform patch testing in the office using the TRUE test (Mekos Laboratories A/S, Hillerod, Denmark). The TRUE test now includes 28 allergens and one control. In the past 2 years, four new allergens were added to the true test: tixocortol pivalate, budesonide, diazolidinyl urea, and imidazolidinyl urea.[65]

The protocol for reading the TRUE test varies among practitioners. According to the TRUE test package insert, results should be interpreted 48 hours after application and then read again at 72 to 96 hours to reduce false-positive and false-negative results. If neomycin or *p*-phenylenediamine allergies are suspected, additional readings at 5 to 7 days may be needed.[66] Some researchers have also found that readings for metals and corticosteroids should also be delayed to 7 days.[67] However, a recent study showed that by delaying readings to 7 days, some reactions to certain fragrances and preservative allergens may dissipate.[68] Therefore, the optimal protocol is probably to read the test on days 3 and 5, and then on day 7 if allergies to metals, topical antibiotics, and PPD are strongly suspected.

According to data from the TRUE test manufacturers, more than one quarter of patients can test positive to one of the TRUE. test allergens.[66] Patients who test negative may be allergic to other substances not included in TRUE test, and therefore require additional testing, often with the more extensive 58-allergen screening series of the North American Contact Dermatitis Group (NACDG). Studies have shown that the TRUE test identifies approximately 70% of clinically relevant allergens when compared with the NACDG panel.[69] For a more individual approach, some patients are tested for a particular assortment of allergens using Finn chambers. In Finn chambers the allergens are applied to filter paper, which is applied to thin 8-mm aluminum disks dispersed in petrolatum.

Once an allergen is identified, patients must be instructed on the importance of strict avoidance. Helpful patient information included in the TRUE test and NACDG series details chemicals and products patients should avoid. Also useful is the contact allergen replacement data (CARD), available to members of the American Contact Dermatitis Society, a resource for physicians that provides safe alternatives to allergens that patients can use.[70] When complete avoidance is impractical, wearing protective barriers can be helpful. For instance, in cases of occupational hand dermatitis, patients can wear protective gloves, ideally vinyl and waterproof, that can be worn atop cotton gloves.[62] However, despite their best efforts at prevention, many patients still present with acute cases of ACD. These outbreaks are often quickly cleared with topical or oral corticosteroids. If they become severe chronic or refractory, patients may need treatment with long-term UVA therapy or immunosuppressive agents such as cyclosporine.

SUMMARY

AD, urticaria, and ACD account for a large percentage of the skin disorders that present at medical offices and emergency departments. With a high degree of morbidity, these diseases can be extremely difficult to manage. Consequently, these diseases continue to be the focus of much of the new research in the field. Recent studies have furthered the understanding of the complex relationship between immune and nonimmune factors in the pathogenesis of these disorders. This research has quickly led to the development of new treatment modalities and protocols for patient care, especially for AD. However, further discovery will be necessary to optimize the management of these often-vexing conditions.

REFERENCES

1. Schulz Larsen F, Hanifin JM. Epidemiology of atopic dermatitis. Immunol Allergy Clin North Am 2002;22:1–24.
2. Simpson EL, Hanifin JM. Atopic dermatitis. Med Clin North Am 2006;90:149–67.
3. Kay J, Gawkrodger DJ, Mortimer MJ, et al. The prevalence of childhood atopic eczema in a general population. J Am Acad Dermatol 1994;30:35–9.
4. Horii KA, Simon SD, Liu DY, et al. Atopic dermatitis in children in the United States, 1997–2004: visit trends, patient and provider characteristics, and prescribing patterns. Pediatrics 2007;120:e527–34.
5. Ben-Gashir MA, Seed PT, Hay PJ. Predictors of atopic dermatitis severity over time. J Am Acad Dermatol 2004;50:349–56.
6. Williams HC, Pembroke AC, Forsdyke H, et al. London-born Caribbean children are at increased risk of atopic dermatitis. J Am Acad Dermatol 1995;32:212–7.
7. Flohr C, Pascoe D, Williams HC. Atopic dermatitis and the "hygiene hypothesis": too clean to be true. Br J Dermatol 2005;15(2):202–16.
8. Sicher SH, Sampson HA. Food hypersensitivity and atopic dermatitis: pathophysiology, epidemiology, diagnosis and management. J Allergy Clin Immunol 1999; 104:S114–22.
9. Jancin B. Antibiotics in infancy up atopic dermatitis risk. Skin Allergy News 2008; 39(8):15.
10. Olesen AB. Role of the early environment for expression of atopic dermatitis. J Am Acad Dermatol 2001;45:S37–40.
11. Williams HC. Atopic dermatitis—the epidemiology, causes and prevention of atopic eczema. Cambridge (UK): Cambridge University Press; 2000.
12. Kang K, Poster AM, Nedorost ST. Atopic dermatitis. In: Bolognia JL, Jorizzo JL, Rapini RP, editors. Dermatology. London: Mosby; 2003. p. 199–214.
13. Eichenfield LF, Hanifin JM, Luger TA, et al. Consensus conference on pediatric atopic dermatitis. J Am Acad Dermatol 2003;49:1088–95.
14. Kang KF, Tian RM. Atopic dermatitis. An evaluation of clinical and laboratory findings. Int J Dermatol 1987;26:27–32.
15. Schultz LF, Holm NV, Henningsen K. Atopic dermatitis: a genetic-epidemiologic study in population-based twin sample. J Am Acad Dermatol 1986;15:487–94.
16. Morar N, Willis-Owen SA, Moffatt MF, et al. The genetics of atopic dermatitis. J Allergy Clin Immunol 2006;118:24–34.

17. Akdis CA, Akdis M, Bieber T, et al. European Academy of Allergology; Clinical Immunology/American Academy of Allergy, Asthma, and Immunology/PRAC-TALL Consensus Group. Diagnosis and treatment of atopic dermatitis in children and adults: European Academy of Allergology; Clinical Immunology/American Academy of Allergy, Asthma, and Immunology/PRACTALL consensus report. Allergy 2006;61:969–87.

18. Novak N, Bieber T, Leung DY. Immune mechanisms leading to atopic dermatitis. J Allergy Clin Immunol 2003;112(6 Suppl):S128–39.

19. The Bantam Medical Dictionary, 7th edition.

20. Sator PG, Schmidt JB, Honigsmann H. Comparison of epidermal hydration and skin surface lipids in healthy individuals and in patients with atopic dermatitis. J Am Acad Dermatol 2003;48:352–8.

21. Hara J, Higuchi K, Okamoto R, et al. High expression of sphingomyelin deacylase is an important determinant of ceramide deficiency leading to barrier disruption in atopic dermatitis. J Invest Dermatol 2000;115:406–13.

22. Sicherer SH, Leung DY. Advances in allergic skin disease, anaphylaxis, and hypersensitivity reactions to foods, drugs, and insects in 2007. J Allergy Clin Immunol 2008;121:1351–8.

23. Howell MD, Kim BE, Gao P, et al. Cytokine modulation of atopic dermatitis filaggrin skin expression. J Allergy Clin Immunol 2007;120:150–5.

24. Kramer MS, Kakuma R. Maternal dietary antigen avoidance during pregnancy and/or lactation for preventing or treating atopic disease in the child. Cochrane Database Syst Rev 2003;(4):CD000133.

25. Hanifin JM, Cooper KD, Ho VC, et al. Guidelines of care for atopic dermatitis. J Am Acad Dermatol 2004;50:391–404.

26. Kalliomaki M, Salmien S, Poussa T, et al. Probiotics and prevention of atopic disease: 4-year follow-up of a randomized placebo-controlled trial. Lancet 2003;361:1869–71.

27. Lee J, Seto D, Bielory L. Meta-analysis of clinical trials of probiotics for prevention and treatment of pediatric atopic dermatitis. J Allergy Clin Immunol 2008;121: 116–21.

28. Nash Karen. Hand dermatitis: determining cause is the first step in treatment. Dermatol Times 2008;60–1.

29. Chamlin SL, Kao J, Frieden IJ, et al. Ceramide dominant barrier repair lipids alleviate childhood atopic dermatitis: changes in barrier function provide a sensitive indicator of disease activity. J Am Acad Dermatol 2002;47:198–208.

30. Sugarman J, Parish LJ. A topical lipid-based barrier repair formulation (EpiCeram cream) is high-effective monotherapy for moderate-to-severe pediatric atopic dermatitis. J Invest Dermatol, in press.

31. Eberlein-Koenig B. Improvement of signs and symptoms in PEA-containing cream-treated adults. Abstract submitted for presentation at: 64th Annual Meeting of the American Academy of Dermatology. San Francisco, March 3–7, 2006.

32. Milgrom H, Berger W, Nayak A, et al. Treatment of childhood asthma with anti-immunoglobulin E antibody (omalizumab). Pediatrics 2001;108(2):E36.

33. Boguniewicz M, Zeichner JA, Eichenfield LF. MAS063DP is effective monotherapy for mild to moderate atopic dermatitis in infants and children: a multicenter, randomized, vehicle-controlled study. J Pediatr 2008;152:854–9.

34. Elias PM, Hatano Y, Williams ML. Basis for the barrier abnormality in atopic dermatitis: Outside-inside-outside pathogenic mechanisms. J Allergy Clin Immunol 2008;121:1337–43.

35. Lipozenčić J, Wolf R. Atopic dermatitis: an update and review of the literature. Dermatol Clin 2007;25:605–12.
36. Tan WP, Goon A, Suresh S. A randomized double-blind controlled trial to compare a triclosan-containing emollient with vehicle for the treatment of atopic dermatitis.
37. Scheinfeld N. Omalizumab: a recombinant humanized monoclonal IgE-blocking antibody. Dermatol Online J 2005;11(1):2.
38. Belloni B, Ziai M, Lim A, et al. Low-dose anti-IgE therapy in patients with atopic eczema with high serum IgE levels. J Allergy Clin Immunol 2007;120:1223–5.
39. Lane JE, Cheyney JM, Lane TN. Treatment of recalcitrant atopic dermatitis with omalizumab. J Am Acad Dermatol 2006;54:68–72.
40. Wendling P. Atopic dermatitis treatments go outside the box. Skin Allergy News 2008;39(10):48.
41. Kimenko T. Whole-body cryotherapy in atopic dermatitis. Arch Dermatol 2008; 144:806–8.
42. Sidbury R. Randomized controlled trial of vitamin D supplementation for winter-related atopic dermatitis in Boston: a pilot study. Br J Dermatol 2008;159(1): 245–7.
43. Beltrani VS. Urticaria and angioedema. Dermatol Clin 1996;14(1):171–98.
44. Soter NA. Acute and chronic urticaria and angioedema. J Am Acad Dermatol 1991;25(1 Pt 2):146–54.
45. Varadarajulu S. Urticaria and angioedema. Controlling acute episodes, coping with chronic cases. Postgrad Med 2005;117(5):25–31.
46. Dibbern DA. Urticaria: selected highlights and recent advances. Med Clin North Am 2006;90:187–209.
47. Tong LJ, Balakrishnan G, Kochan JP, et al. Assessment of autoimmunity in patients with chronic urticaria. J Allergy Clin Immunol 1997;99(4):461–5.
48. Kaplan AP. Chronic urticaria: pathogenesis and treatment. J Allergy Clin Immunol 2004;114:465–74.
49. Kennedy MS. Evaluation of chronic eczema and urticaria and angioedema. Immunol Allergy Clin North Am 1999;19:19–33.
50. Kaplan AP. Clinical practice. Chronic urticaria and angioedema. N Engl J Med 2002;346:175–9.
51. Komarow HD, Metcalfe DD. Office-based management of urticaria. Am J Med 2008;121:379–84.
52. Kozel MMA, Boussuyt PMM, Mekkes JR, et al. Laboratory tests and identified diagnoses in patients with physical and chronic urticaria and angioedema: a systematic review. J Am Acad Dermatol 2003;48:409–16.
53. Champion RH, Roberts SOB, Carpenter RG, et al. Urticaria and angio-edema: a review of 554 patients. Br J Dermatol 2004;29:217–21.
54. Kozel MM, Mekkes JR, Bossuyt PM, et al. The effectiveness of a history-based diagnostic approach in chronic urticaria and angioedema. Arch Dermatol 1998; 134:1575–80.
55. Sabroe RA, Grattan CE, Francis DM, et al. The autologous serum skin test: a screening test for autoantibodies in chronic idiopathic urticaria. Br J Dermatol 1999;140:446–52.
56. Brunetti L, Francavilla R, Miniello VL, et al. High prevalence of autoimmune urticaria in children with chronic urticaria. J Allergy Clin Immunol 2004;114:922–7.
57. Worcester S. New advances refine chronic urticaria screening. Skin Allergy News 2008;39(4):14.
58. Cox L, Li JT, Nelson H, et al. Allergen immunotherapy: a practice parameter second update. J Allergy Clin Immunol 2007;120(3 Suppl):S25–85.

59. Siebenhaar F. High-dose desloratadine decreases wheal volume and improves cold provocation thresholds compared with standard-dose treatment in patients with acquired cold urticaria: a randomized, placebo-controlled, crossover study. J Allergy Clin Immunol 2009;123:672–9.

60. Simons FER. Advances in H1-antihistamines. N Engl J Med 2004;351:2203–17.

61. Beltrani VS, Beltrani VP. Contact dermatitis. Ann Allergy Asthma Immunol 1997; 78:160–75.

62. Mark BJ, Slavin RG. Allergic contact dermatitis. Med Clin North Am 2006;90: 169–85.

63. Peate WF. Occupational skin disease. Am Fam Physician 2002;66:1025–32.

64. Rietschel RL, Fowler JR. Fisher's contact dermatitis. 5th edition. Philadelphia: Lippincott Williams & Wilkins; 2001.

65. Andersen KE, Paulsen E. Concordance of patch test results with four new TRUE test allergens compared with the same allergens from Chemotechnique. Contact dermatitis 2009;60:59.

66. T.R.U.E. Test. Available at: http://www.truetest.com/. Accessed April 2, 2009.

67. Geier J, Gefeller O, Wiechmann K, et al. Patch test reactions at D4, D5, D6. Contact dermatitis 1999;40:119–26.

68. Davis MDP, Bhate K, Rohlinger AL, et al. Delayed patch test reading after 5 days: the Mayo Clinic experience. J Am Acad Dermatol 2008;59:225–33.

69. Larkin A, Rietschel RL. The utility of patch tests using larger screening series of allergens. Am J Contact Dermatitis 1998;9:142–5.

70. Gillete B. Keeping pace with allergens: investigators find new triggers for contact dermatitis. Dermatol Times 2008;59.

Pigmentary Disorders

Paul T. Rose, MD, JD

KEYWORDS

- Pigmentary disorders • Melanocytes • Vitiligo
- Pityriasis alba • Tuberous sclerosis • Café au lait spots
- Tinea versicolor • Melasma • Fixed drug reaction
- Postinflammatory pigmentation

Pigmentary disorders are frequently encountered in the practice of adult medicine. Patients routinely present with concerns about areas of pigment, pigment change or lesions that have changed in color. Other times it is the clinician who notices an area(s) of pigment or pigment change.

For the most part these disorders are rarely associated with systemic disease but at times alterations of pigment can signify severe disease. In addition, although changes in pigment may only be cosmetic, such alterations can also be a source of discomfort and great emotional stress for patients.

It is important for physicians practicing internal medicine and family practice to be familiar with some of the more common disorders that may present in the course of practice. The clinician needs to be able to recognize situations in which a pigmentary alteration suggests serious disease such as underlying malignancy. In these instances, an examination and laboratory evaluation should be commensurate with the possibility of these diseases.

In this article, the more common presentations of pigmentary disorders in the adult population are discussed. There are several pediatric genetic conditions associated with pigmentary disease that are complicated by systemic disease and other medical problems. The clinician is referred to the pediatric literature to review these entities.

MELANOCYTES AND MELANOCYTE FUNCTION

A primary function of melanin is protection from ultraviolet (UV) light. It is produced by cells derived from the neural crest referred to as melanocytes. Melanocytes exist in the skin, retina, stria vascularis of the ear, leptomeninges, and hair matrix. These cells possess the melanosomes responsible for the production of melanin. The melanosomes contain tyrosinase, which is utilized to convert tyrosine to melanin.[1] In the skin, melanosomes are transferred from the melanocytes to groups of keratinocytes where they provide color for skin.

Academic Alliance in Dermatology, 4238 West Kennedy Boulevard, Tampa, FL 33609, USA
E-mail address: paultrose@yahoo.com

Med Clin N Am 93 (2009) 1225–1239
doi:10.1016/j.mcna.2009.08.005
0025-7125/09/$ – see front matter © 2009 Elsevier Inc. All rights reserved.

Two forms of melanin exist: eumelanin and pheomelanin. Eumelanin produces the brown pigmentation of the skin, whereas pheomelanin produces more of a yellow and red coloration.

There is no appreciable difference in the number of melanocytes between whites, Asians and African Americans. Differences exist in the amount of melanization in melanosomes, number, and distribution of melanosomes. In addition, melanosomes are smaller in whites than in African Americans.[2]

Pigmentary disorders occur for various reasons such as loss of melanocytes, increase or decrease in melanocyte activity. The pigmentary disorders are commonly divided into 2 broad categories: those of increased pigmentation (hyperpigmentation) and those of decreased pigmentation (hypopigmentation).

DISORDERS OF DECREASED PIGMENTATION
Vitiligo

One of the most frequently noticed disorders of pigmentation is vitiligo. Vitiligo is characterized by discrete areas of skin and mucous membranes that have lost pigment. This loss of pigment can be localized or generalized. The disease tends to be progressive and can be emotionally disabling to patients. The occurrence of vitiligo is estimated to be approximately 1% in the United States and ranges from 0.5% to 2% worldwide.[3,4] The disease tends to occur between the ages of 10 and 30 years and rarely occurs in infants or in the elderly.

The cause of vitiligo is unclear but various theories exist as to why melanocytes are lost. It seems that there are genetic and nongenetic aspects to the acquisition of the disease. A family history of the disorder exists in 30% of patients.[2] It is speculated that vitiligo is primarily an autoimmune process.[5-8] Vitiligo is associated with other diseases of an autoimmune etiology.

Other diseases with well-documented autoimmune etiologies that have been associated with vitiligo include alopecia areata, Hashimoto thyroiditis, Graves' disease, Addison's disease, uveitis, chronic mucocutaneous candidiasis, autoimmune polyglandular syndrome, pernicious anemia, inflammatory bowel disease, psoriasis, and insulin-dependent diabetes.[9] It is estimated that almost 30% of vitiligo patients have thyroid disease.[10]

Other mechanisms cited as possible causes of the loss of melanocytes in vitiligo include cytotoxic factors, neural factors,[11] alterations in melanocyte function,[12] and possibly factors related to oxidant and antioxidant reactions.[13]

Vitiligo can be divided into 4 variations referred to as generalized, localized or segmental, universal, and acrofacial. The generalized type tends to be relatively symmetric and the macules and patches tend to have well-circumscribed borders. The areas of depigmentation appear to expand in a centrifugal manner and the progression of the disease is generally slow.

The most commonly affected sites include the dorsal hands, face, neck, body creases, axillae, scalp and genitalia (**Figs. 1** and **2**). Areas of depigmentation often occur at orifices such as the nostrils, mouth and anus. Other common areas of involvement include the nipples and umbilicus. These patients may also have a higher incidence of halo nevi.

Patients with the generalized form are more likely to have an associated autoimmune or endocrine disease. The localized form may be asymmetric and may follow a dermatomal distribution. It tends to be more common in children than the generalized form and has been found to be more difficult to treat. The occurrence of autoimmune disease is less in this form of vitiligo. These patients may demonstrate

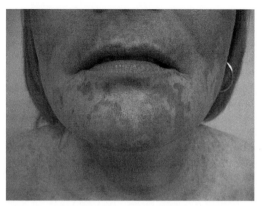

Fig. 1. Generalized vitiligo. The loss of pigment in the perioral area is common.

organ specific antibodies and they have a diminished response to psoralens and UVA light (PUVA) compared with patients with the more generalized type of vitiligo.

As with some other dermatologic diseases such as psoriasis and lichen planus, vitiligo can be spread by the Koebner phenomenon. The Koebner phenomenon is the initiation of new lesions or points of involvement that occur as a result of trauma, particularly mechanical trauma such as scratching. With vitiligo the areas most likely to be affected include the elbows, other areas of bony prominences and areas of sunburn.

On clinical examination, the physician will notice macules and patches of decreased or totally absent pigment. At times the areas may appear erythematous or have an erythematous border, which may indicate an ongoing inflammatory process. The patient may present with concerns about obvious areas of pigment loss but there

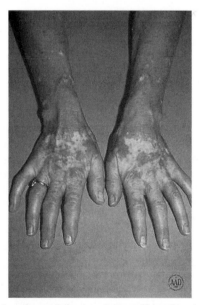

Fig. 2. Vitiligo. The dorsal surface of the hands are affected and the involvement is fairly symmetric. (*Reproduced with permission from* the American Academy of Dermatology, Copyright © 2009. All rights reserved.)

may be areas that are not so easily apparent. This is particularly true in patients who are light complected.[14]

The use of a Woods light (UV light in the range of 320–400 nm) can greatly assist in locating areas of pigment disruption.[15] Examination with the Woods light can reveal areas of hypopigmentation. A complete examination should include inspection of the genitalia and areas of skin folds as these areas can be easily overlooked.

The patient should be questioned as to any history of related disorders such as thyroid disease or autoimmune conditions. It may be prudent to test for thyroid function including thyrotropin, antithyroglobulin, antithyroid peroxidase antibodies, thyroid-stimulating hormone (TSH), free T4, free T3. An antinuclear antibody test may be helpful in assessing autoimmune status. Other tests may include glucose and glycosylated hemoglobin. Because the eyes can be affected by vitiligo, an ophthalmologic examination should be considered.

To confirm the diagnosis a punch biopsy can be taken. A 3-mm biopsy from the border of the lesion such that it includes pigmented and nonpigmented skin can be helpful. Histologic examination reveals an absence of melanocytes and loss of epidermal pigmentation.[16]

As mentioned earlier there are multiple diseases that can be associated with vitiligo. In the adult patient the clinician should be aware of the association of vitiligo with uveitis, aseptic meningitis, dysacusia, tinnitus, poliosis, and alopecia. These are the features of Vogt Koyanagi syndrome.[17]

Another syndrome that includes vitiligo is Alezzandrini syndrome. Patients with this disorder have facial vitiligo, poliosis, deafness, unilateral visual changes, and decreased visual acuity.[17]

Although the diagnosis of vitiligo may be obvious when there are extensive areas of pigment loss, there are instances where the diagnosis can be less obvious. The differential diagnosis can include tinea versicolor, idiopathic guttate hypomelanosis, postinflammatory hypopigmenation, halo nevi, and regressing melanoma.

The treatment of vitiligo is based on finding ways to stimulate melanocytes, stopping the destruction of melanocytes and providing ways to allow for melanocyte migration/population of areas. For the areas to repigment, the melanocytes must come from pilosebaceous units and the remaining melanocytes at the edges of lesions.

Successful treatment of vitiligo often depends on early intervention. Even then the results can be less than optimal. Clinicians must remember that the disease can cause marked stress for patients. It can be disfiguring and patients may benefit from psychological therapy.

Numerous treatments are available. In most instances the patient will benefit from consultation with a dermatologist experienced in the various regimens available. Possible treatments can include the use of potent steroids applied locally; however, there is a risk of steroid atrophy. If the response is not fairly brisk, the patient may need to consider more aggressive therapy. Some dermatologists have recommended tacrolimus 0.03%–0.1% topically. Tacrolimus has been used primarily for head and neck involvement.[18] The use of UV light can be beneficial. A common regimen is the use of narrow band UVB, which is considered safe for children, pregnant women, and lactating women.[19] This may be combined with narrowband UVB.[20] PUVA can be helpful and in some studies as many as 70% of patients showed significant improvement but this was after a period of 12 to 24 months and 150 treatments. Many patients decline such frequent treatments especially when no permanent cure can be provided.[21] Some dermatologists recommend the drug psoralen with sunlight, which allows for greater treatment flexibility for the patient but the patient may be more subject to sunburn from inaccurate dosing of UV light. The use of the excimer laser has been shown to provide a response to vitiligo. The laser uses monochromatic light at 308 nm.[22] There have been reports of positive responses with the combination of tacrolimus and excimer laser.[23]

In many cases the response is less than satisfactory and patients may want to consider the use of camouflage agents or in severe cases, the use of a depigmenting chemical to totally and permanently eliminate the areas of remaining pigment. Depigmentation can be accomplished with 20% monobenzone. This treatment is generally reserved for patients with at least 50% involvement[24] because of the increased risk of skin cancer. Patients with vitiligo should be advised to use UVA/UVB sunscreen.

Pityriasis Alba

Pityriasis alba is a common dermatologic disorder in children. It is usually evident before puberty and most of these patients first present to pediatricians or dermatologists with a facial rash. The typical lesions of pityriasis alba are hypopigmented patches or macules with slight scale, primarily on the face and less frequently the neck, trunk, and extremities (**Fig. 3**). Although the cause is unclear, these patients often have a history of atopy.[25,26] The patients may not have clear evidence of atopic dermatitis but they often have environmental allergies signified by nasal rhinitis.[27]

Pityriasis alba does not create any permanent damage to the skin, however parents and patients are often troubled by the uneven pigmentation. The differential diagnosis may include tinea versicolor and vitiligo. Tinea versicolor can be ruled out with a KOH or chlorazole preparation. Unlike tinea versicolor or pityriasis alba, vitiligo does not scale and the loss of pigment with vitiligo is complete and well demonstrated with a Woods lamp examination.

Treatment of pityriasis alba often includes the use of lubricants and mild topical steroids. Steroids of class V or sometimes class IV are favored. The problem can be chronic in childhood and often improves after puberty.

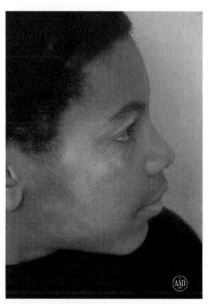

Fig. 3. Pityriasis alba. Patchy areas of decreased pigment. Patients frequently have a history of allergies. (*Reproduced with permission from* the American Academy of Dermatology, Copyright © 2009. All rights reserved.)

Idiopathic Guttate Hypomelanosis

A common complaint of adult patients is the occurrence of depigmented macules particularly on the arms and legs. These irregularly shaped macules are most common in light-skinned individuals who have had a marked sun exposure and they are more common in women.[4] The lesions are devoid of melanocytes and this seems to be related to the destruction of melanocytes over time (**Fig. 4**).[28] Treatment of this disorder is limited. Cryotherapy and camouflage makeup may be helpful. Some patients may use dihydroxyacetone preparations to hide the areas. It is important to stress to patients that the lesions are harmless. The use of sunscreens is recommended as these areas of depigmentation may be more susceptible to skin cancer.

Postinflammatory Hypopigmentation

Many inflammatory conditions can alter melanocyte function leading to changes in localized areas of pigmentation, which can be hyper- or hypopigmented. These alterations in pigment are more evident in patients who are darker complected, particularly Hispanics, African Americans, and those of Middle Eastern ethnicity.[25]

Frequent causes of postinflammatory pigmentation include trauma, discoid lupus, sarcoid, chemical irritation, or burn. Areas of skin that are repeatedly rubbed can develop hyperpigmentation. This is commonly observed in athletes who wear helmets and subsequently have areas of hyperpigmentation along the forehead where the helmet rubs against the skin.

Clinicians sometimes see patients with type IV to VI skin who present with a complaint of hypopigmentation following treatment with lasers, chemical peels, and intense pulse light devices. Hypopigmentation may also result from the use of freezing treatments with liquid nitrogen or other cold-producing compounds. Similarly treatment with cautery devices can leave hypopigmented areas. Another commonly observed source of hypopigmentation is acne. The acne lesions may resolve but the inflammatory reaction may cause a change in melanocyte function leading to hypopigmentation in the area of the lesions.

Tuberous Sclerosis

Tuberous sclerosis is a congenital disease characterized by seizures, mental retardation, and adenoma sebaceum.[25] Patients often have hypopigmented macules located on the arms, legs, and trunk but they may be located anywhere. These lesions are a key finding in tuberous sclerosis and may be the first clinical signs of the disease.

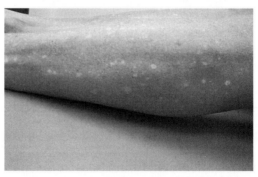

Fig. 4. Idiopathic guttate hypomelanosis. Patients are often fair skinned and have a history of chronic sun exposure.

The lesions are termed ash leaf or lance ovate hypopigmented macules (**Fig. 5**). Typically the shape is pointed at 1 pole and broad at the opposite end resembling the ash leaf. The macules are usually 1 to 3 cm in diameter and can vary in number from 1 to 30 plus lesion(s). It is thought that between 40% and 90% of patients have these ash leaf macules.[29] Other skin manifestations of the disease include angiofibromas, fibrous plaques and periungual and subungual fibromas.

The ash leaf macules can be confused with vitiligo but, unlike vitiligo, there is not a total loss of pigment. These areas of decreased pigment are stable and do not expand, whereas vitiligo lesions often expand with time and the affected areas tend to be symmetric. When a clinician observes 3 or more of these ash leaf lesions, a possible diagnosis of tuberous sclerosis should be considered.

Tinea Versicolor

Tinea versicolor is a ubiquitous skin disease. Patients often notice the pigment changes during the summer months and may refer to the areas of decreased pigment as "sun spots." This disorder presents as macules and patches of decreased pigment associated with a fine scale. The lesions tend to be round or scalloped in shape (**Fig. 6**). The affected areas are usually not symptomatic but, on occasion, patients may complain of itching. A variant of tinea versicolor may produce increased pigmentation.

Tinea versicolor is infectious and is caused by a yeast termed *Malessezia furfur*.[30,31] This yeast is a normal component of skin flora. As with other yeasts, it flourishes in an environment of heat, darkness, and moisture. It frequently appears on the trunk and arms and is rarely seen on the face. The areas affected seem to be areas of higher sebaceous activity and associated higher lipid content. In some instances the presentation may involve the body creases or it may be more follicular. The follicular form may demonstrate pustules and papules. Tinea versicolor is more prevalent in the 15- to 35-year-old age group.

Other diseases have been associated with tinea versicolor. These include Cushing's syndrome, hyperhidrosis, and altered immune status such as HIV.[32]

The yeast has the ability to alter melanocyte metabolism by producing dicarboxylic acids that inhibit the activity of tyrosinase thus causing a decrease in pigmentation.[32] Although the yeast may exist in everyone, some people are more prone to its effects.

Tinea versicolor can be confused with vitiligo but the confusion can be eliminated when the clinician considers that tinea versicolor usually has scales. A KOH or

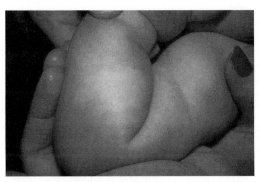

Fig. 5. Ash leaf macule. (*Reproduced with permission from* the American Academy of Dermatology, Copyright © 2009. All rights reserved.)

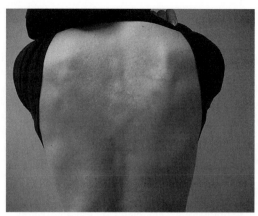

Fig. 6. Tinea versicolor. Affected areas may have fine loose scale referred to as "furfuraceous" scale. A diagnostic clue is the ability to loosen the scale by gentle scratching of the involved area. This is referred to as the "scratch sign."

chlorazole preparation can be used to demonstrate the yeast forms microscopically. Typically the clinician will see what is referred to as "spaghetti and meatballs," the combination of short, relatively straight rods that represent the "spaghetti" and the often associated round spores that represent the "meatballs."

At times there is a lack of scale and the clinician may still consider the possibility of vitiligo. Use of a Wood's lamp will show that with vitiligo there is a total loss of pigment in the affected areas, whereas there will be some pigment still evident in areas of tinea versicolor.

Tinea versicolor can be treated but it commonly recurs, particularly in the warmer months. Various treatment protocols exist.[33] If the patient prefers to rely on topical therapy, selenium sulfide lotion 2.5% can be used. Patients should also use a shampoo containing selenium sulfide or ketoconazole to eradicate any yeast that may be present in the hair and scalp. Other topical treatments include the use of antifungals such as ketoconazole, clotrimazole, tolnaftate, and other similar compounds.

Most patients prefer a single course of oral antifungals.[34] A common treatment regimen is the use of ketoconazole 400 mg a day for 2 days. The patient is advised to exercise after taking the medication to allow for enhanced distribution. Some physicians repeat the course in a week. Other variations include the use of ketoconazole 200 mg daily for 1 week.

Although there is some concern about the use of ketoconazole and other oral antifungals in regard to liver function, such short courses of therapy are rarely associated with hepatic disease. Patients should be questioned on any history of liver disease and use of alcohol. It is important that patients' avoid alcohol use while on these systemic antifungal medications.

No matter which course of therapy is selected it is important to inform patients that the areas of altered pigment may persist for several months until the melanocyte function is restored.

DISORDERS OF HYPERPIGMENTATION
Melasma

Probably the most frequent complaint from female patients regarding pigment change concerns increased facial pigmentation. This pigment change is often caused by melasma. Melasma is an acquired condition characterized by dark brown colored, well-demarcated patches that often localize to sun-exposed areas such as the malar eminence, upper lip, forehead, neck, and chin (**Fig. 7**). On occasion it can be present on the arms. It is more frequently observed in type IV to VI Fitzpatrick skin types and occurs more commonly in young women.

Melasma commonly affects women in the second or third trimester of pregnancy and is often called the "mask of pregnancy." It usually recedes after delivery and may increase with subsequent pregnancies. Men can be affected and it is estimated that they account for perhaps 10% of cases.[4]

Apart from pregnancy this disorder can also be caused by the use of birth control pills, which essentially mimic pregnancy .Other causes include medications such as phenytoin, hepatic disease, endocrine disorders. In some cases no clear cause is evident. Many clinicians believe that estrogen may be an important factor in causing melasma, the fact that postmenopausal women taking estrogen do not get melasma would suggest otherwise.[32]

On physical examination, there is usually a tan to brown pigment pattern but the pigment may also have a bluish appearance. The tan brown color suggests epidermal pigmentation, whereas the bluish color suggests dermal deposition. Epidermal pigment is more amenable to treatment than dermal pigment.

Melasma during pregnancy generally improves after the pregnancy. The treatment of melasma associated with the use of birth control pills and other causes can often be frustrating. Although it is often possible to improve melasma, a total cure can be difficult. Treatment is usually based on topical therapy, which includes the use of a bleaching cream with a hydroquinone.[35–39] Hydroquinones work by limiting the conversion of dopa to melanin via the action of tyrosinase. Treatment may be enhanced with the use of a retinoid such as tretinoin and possibly a low dose steroid to decrease the inflammatory response. When using a bleaching cream, it is important to advise patients to try a test area before full application as some patients experience an allergic or irritant reaction. Patients should be advised that application to areas of normal skin may result in hypopigmentation of these unintended areas. In rare instances, hydroquinones can cause ochronosis in African Americans, which produces a reticulated pattern of pigmentation on the face.[40]

Other medications used to reduce melasma include azeleic acid, kogic acid, and the α-hydroxy acids, licorice extract, and various peels. Some physicians are now using

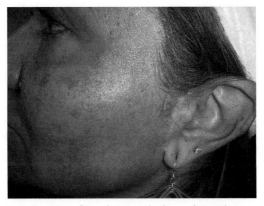

Fig. 7. Melasma. A common area of involvement is the malar eminence.

various lasers and intense pulsed light (IPL) to treat melasma.[41] The lasers that have been used include the erbium YAG, Q switched Ruby laser, Q switched neodynium YAG, Q switched Alexandrite, and the CO_2 laser.[33]

Patients must also be advised that sun exposure exacerbates the condition. Physicians should stress to patients the need to use sunscreens that block UVA and UVB light.

Fixed Drug Reaction

Some patients have an allergic reaction to medication that produces pigmented areas. The affected areas are most commonly solitary but can be multiple and are often discoid in shape. They frequently occur on the trunk, genitalia, and oral mucosa.[32] Patients often complain of itching in the area involved. The morphology can vary greatly ranging from macules to vesiculobullous lesions. Typically, lesions tend to appear in the same location on re-exposure to the offending medication. The drug reaction often occurs within 8 hours in patients who are already sensitized. In some instances, a reaction can be delayed for several weeks from the time of taking the substance.

Frequent causes of fixed drug reactions include minocyline, tetracycline, aspirin, nonsteroid anti-inflammatory drugs, trimethoprim, sulfmethoxazole, barbiturates, acetaminophen, hydroxyzine, and celecoxib.[42,43] Many other drugs and various Asian herbal preparations have been linked to fixed drug reactions.

Treatment is based on removal of the causative agent and the use of a mid- to high-potency topical steroid depending on the area affected. In some instances, the use of oral steroids may be warranted. If the pruritus is severe, an antihistamine can also be used.

Systemic Diseases Associated with Pigment Change

On occasion a patient may present with concerns about diffuse darkening of skin similar to a tan but without a significant history of sun exposure. Such a change in pigment should cause the physician to consider the possibility of hemochromatosis, Addison's disease and possibly metastatic melanoma. Although one might imagine that such patients would have other signs and symptoms that prompted a previous medical evaluation, such patients often present with the alteration in skin color as the primary symptom.

Hemochromatosis is an iron storage disease, most importantly involving the liver. These patients have a brown gray pigmentation that is most evident in sun-exposed areas such as the face, arms, and hands. Pigmentation may also be present at the mucous membranes. Hemochromatosis is more common in men and often evident between the ages of 30 and 50 years. Patients with hemochromatosis are at risk of developing cirrhosis and hepatocellular cancer. Other associated diseases include diabetes arthropathy and cardiac problems.[17,44] Patients have elevated levels of serum iron, ferritin, and iron-binding protein. Treatment is largely based on phlebotomy to reduce iron levels.

Addison's disease affects the adrenal gland resulting in adrenal insufficiency. In affecting the adrenal glands, melanocyte function is also affected. Patients present with a diffuse pattern of pigmentation that primarily involves sun-exposed areas but areas the inguinal area and axillae may also be affected.[17] Patients may notice an increase in pigment of nevi, hair, and nails. Along with pigmentary changes, patients may experience fatigue, weight loss, and abdominal symptoms.

Biliary cirrhosis can also be accompanied by diffuse brown black alteration in skin color. Other manifestations may include marked pruritus and jaundice. Some patients may have an area on the back with no pigment change. The disease has a poor prognosis as patients often develop esophageal varices and hepatic failure.

Acanthosis Nigricans

Acanthosis nigricans is a common skin condition frequently observed in African Americans. The physical appearance is that of symmetric, darkened areas of skin that are thickened and described as "velvety" in texture, and located in areas of creases such as the axillae, neck, and groin (**Fig. 8**). Other locations include the face, elbows, knees, and hands.[45,46]

Acanthosis nigricans can be divided into 3 types. Type I is associated with malignant disease. Type II is familial and type III is associated with obesity, insulin-resistant disorders and other endocrine disorders.[47] Type III acanthosis nigricans is the most common form of the disorder. Of those cases, most are related to obesity without other related diseases. As discussed earlier type III acanthosis nigricans can be associated with endocrine disorders including diabetes mellitus, Cushing's disease, Addison's disease, pinealoma, and hyperandrogenic and hypogonadal states.

Some medications have been linked to the development of acanthosis nigricans including oral contraceptives, insulin, glucocorticoids, nicotinic acid, triazinate, methyltestosterone, and pituitary extracts.[46] The familial form is inherited as an autosomal dominant and is usually apparent at birth but may develop later in childhood. There are instances when acanthosis nigricans can be a clue to serious underlying disease. In particular, acanthosis nigricans can be associated with stomach cancer and lung carcinoma.[47] A thorough history, examination, appropriate laboratory workup, and radiologic studies may provide clues to an undetected malignancy. An extensive workup may be required particularly when a patient presents with sudden onset of acanthosis nigricans.

Treatment of this disorder is based primarily on removing the cause. In the case of underlying malignancy, detecting and removing the malignancy can lead to improvement in the condition. Control of an underlying endocrine disorder may help patients with type III acanthosis nigricans. Loss of weight can produce improvement in patients who have acanthosis nigricans type III as a result of obesity.

Some patients have benefited from medications such as metformin, oral isotretinoin, topical retinoic acid, topical salicylic acid, and oral fish oil. Successes have been reported with the CO_2 laser and the long-pulsed Alexandrite laser.[48]

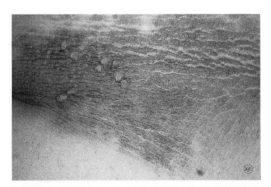

Fig. 8. Acanthosis nigricans. Areas of creases are usually involved and have a "velvety" texture. (*Reproduced with permission from* the American Academy of Dermatology, Copyright © 2009. All rights reserved.)

Postinflammatory Hyperpigmentation

As with postinflammatory hypopigmentation some patients, particularly patients with Fitzpatrick type IV to VI skin types, tend to produce increased pigment with inflammatory skin disorders. For reasons that are not entirely clear the inflammatory process may cause an increase in melanocyte activity or deposition of melanin into the dermis. The physician can differentiate the location of the pigment with a Woods light. With the Wood's light, epidermal pigmentation is enhanced, whereas with dermal deposition the pigment is not highlighted. Treatment should be focused on the cause of the inflammatory process. Hydroquinone preparations can be helpful. Some physicians have had limited success with lasers and various chemical peels.

Café au Lait Spots

Café au lait macules are common. These are well-demarcated macules with increased pigment and irregular borders that vary widely in size (**Fig. 9**). They are often observed on the trunk and extremities and can often be seen at birth. The importance of café au lait spots is the association with neurofibromatosis.[25] Neurofibromatosis is a neurocutaneous disease. Type I (Von Recklinghausen disease) accounts for more than 85% of cases and is an autosomal dominant form affecting chromosome 17. It occurs in approximately 1 in 3500 births.[49,50]

Although the finding of a café au lait spot or even a few can be observed in normal children, the finding of 6 or more café au lait macules occurs in more than 60% of patients with type I neurofibromatosis. The finding of 6 or more café au lait spots greater than 1.5 cm in diameter is considered diagnostic for neurofibromatosis.[51] Children may be born with hypertelorism, low set ears, and macrocephaly. Patients may also have sacral hypertrichosis, cutis vertices gyrate, macroglossia, giant pigmented hairy nevi, and Lisch nodules in the irides.

Type I patients often develop axillary freckling (Crowe sign), which is characteristic of type I and observed in 20% to 50% of patients. Type I patients develop various types of neurofibromas. These lesions appear as papules or nodules that have a soft or rubbery consistency and may have a bluish-pink hue. Plexiform neurofibromas are common. These are subcutaneous nodules that are comprised of multiple encapsulated neurofibromas. Type I patients are at a markedly increased risk of developing a malignancy. The risk for malignant myeloid disease in children is approximately 200 to 500 times greater than in age-matched controls.[52]

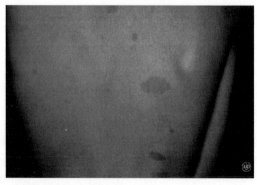

Fig. 9. Café au lait spots. Six or more of these lesions greater than 1.5 cm are diagnostic of neurofibromatosis.

Type II neurofibromatosis is caused by a defect in chromosome 22.[53] These patients are less likely to have skin lesions but characteristically have acoustic neuromas. They may have presenile posterior cortical cataracts and malignant tumors of the central nervous system. These patients rarely have more than 5 café au lait spots and rarely have plexiform neuromas or axillary freckling. They may have skin lesions that are neurofibromas or schwannomas. The lesions are superficial and comprised of papules that may be hypertrichotic and have a rough texture.

Two other forms of neurofibromatosis are described. Type III is a mixed form and type IV is akin to type II but has cutaneous neurofibromas.

SUMMARY

A large number of pigmentary disorders exist and although not all dermatologic entities are covered in this article, some of the pigmentary disorders that an internist or general practitioner is likely to encounter are reviewed. The clinician must be able to recognize pigmentary changes that suggest a serious underlying disease. In a situation where a malignancy or other serious illness may exist, an extensive evaluation to detect the disorder is required. This approach can allow for early treatment and referral to an appropriate specialist if necessary. The clinician must also recognize that pigmentary disorders that are essentially cosmetic still cause concern for the patient and can be emotionally distressing. These patients need emotional support and in some cases referral to a mental health specialist.

REFERENCES

1. Jimbow K, Quevedo WC Jr, Prota G, et al. Biology of melanocyte disorders. In: Freedberg IM, Eisen AZ, Wolff K, et al, editors. Fitzpatrick's dermatology in general medicine. 5th edition. New York: McGraw-Hill; 1999.
2. Boissy RE. The melanocyte: its structure, function and subpopulations in skin, eyes and hair. Dermatol Clin 1988;6:161–73.
3. Lerner AB, Norland JJ. Vitiligo: the loss of pigment in skin, hair and eyes. J Dermatol 1978;5:1–8.
4. Disturbances of pigmentation. In: James WD, Bergen TG, Elston DM, editors. Andrews textbook of dermatology. 10th edition. Philadelphia: Saunders, Elsevier; 2006. p. 853–68.
5. Le Poole IC, Luiten RM. Autoimmune etiology of generalized vitiligo. Curr Dir Autoimmun 2008;10:227–43.
6. Ongennae K, Van Geel N, Naeyaert JM. Evidence for an autoimmune pathogenesis of vitiligo. Pigment Cell Res 2003;16:90–100.
7. Schallreuter KU, Wood JM, Phtelkow MR, et al. Regulation of melanin biosynthesis in the human epidermis tetrahydrobiopterin. Science 1994;263(5152): 1444–6.
8. Mollet I, Ongenae K, Naeyaert JM. Origin, clinical presentation and diagnosis of hypomelanotic skin disorders. Dermatol Clin 2007;25:363–71.
9. Bologna JL, Pawelek JM. Biology of hypopigmentation. J Am Acad Dermatol 1988;19:217–25.
10. Cunliffe WJ, Hall R, Newell DJ, et al. Vitiligo, thyroid diseases and autoimmunity. Br J Dermatol 1968;80:135–9.
11. Gauthier Y, Andre M, Taieb A. A clinical appraisal of vitiligo theories: is melanocyte loss a melanocytorrhagy. Pigment Cell Res 2003;16:322–32.
12. Njoo MD, Westerhof W. Vitiligo: pathogenesis and treatment. Am J Clin Dermatol 2001;2:167–81.

13. Ortonne J. Vitiligo and disorders of hypopigmentation. In: Bolognia U, Jorizzo J, Rapini R, editors, Dermatology, vol. 1, 2nd edition, Spain: Elsevier; 2008. p. 947–74.
14. Drake L, Dinehart SM, Farmer ER, et al. Guidelines of care for vitiligo. J Am Acad Dermatol 1996;35:620–6.
15. Asawananda P, Taylor CR. Wood's light in dermatology. Int J Dermatol 1999;38:801–7.
16. Spielvogel RL, Kantor RL. Pigmentary disorders of the skin. In: Elder DE, Elenitsas R, Jaworsky C, et al. Lever's histopathology of the skin. 8th edition. Philadelphia: Lippincott Williams & Wilkins; 1997. p. 617–23.
17. Mosher DB, Fitzpatrick TB, Ortonne JP, et al. Hypomelanoses and hypermelanoses. In: Freedberg IM, Eisen AZ, Wolff K, et al, editors. Fitzpatrick's dermatology in general medicine. 5th edition. New York: McGraw-Hill; 1999. p. 945–1017.
18. Grimes PE, Soriano T, Dytoc MT, et al. Topical tacrolimus therapy for vitiligo: therapeutic responses and skin messenger RNA expression of proinflammatory cytokines. J Am Acad Dermatol 2004;51:52–61.
19. Hercogova J, Buggiani G, Prignanano F, et al. Rational approach to the treatment of vitiligo and other hypomelanoses. Dermatol Clin 2007;25:383–92.
20. Esfandiarpour I, Ekhlasi A, Frajzadeh S, et al. The efficacy of picrolimus 1% cream plus narrow band ultraviolet B in the treatment of vitiligo: a double blind placebo controlled clinical trial. J Dermatolog Treat 2008;20:14–8.
21. Habif T. Clinical dermatology: a color guide to diagnosis and therapy. In: Light related diseases and disorders of pigmentation. 2nd edition. St. Louis (MO): C.V. Mosby Company; 1989. p. 488–97.
22. Esposito M, Soda R, Costanzo A, et al. Treatment of vitiligo with the 308 nm excimer laser. Clin Exp Dermatol 2004;29:133–7.
23. Lotti T, Prignano F, Buggiani G. New and experimental treatment of vitiligo and other hypomelanoses. Dermatol Clin 2007;25(3):393–400.
24. Canizares O, Jaramilla FU, Kerdel Vegas F. Leukomelanoderma subsequent to the application of monobenzylether of hydroquinone. Arch Dermatol 1958;77:220–3.
25. Paller AS, Mancini AJ, editors. Eczematous eruptions in childhood, Hurwitz clinical pediatric dermatology. 3rd edition. Philadelphia: Elsevier Saunders; 2006. p. 49–84.
26. Wells BT, Whyte HJ, Kierland RR. Pityriasis alba: a ten year survey and review of the literature. Arch Dermatol 1960;82:183–9.
27. Blessman Weber M, Sponchiado de Avilla LG, Albaneze R, et al. Pityriasis alba: a study of pathogenic factors. J Eur Acad Dermatol Venereol 2002;16:463–8.
28. Wallace ML, Grichnik JM, Prieto VG, et al. Numbers and differentiation status of melanocytes in idiopathic guttate hypomelanosis. J Cutan Pathol 1998;25:375–9.
29. Fitzpatrick TB, Szabo G, Hori Y, et al. White leaf shaped macules. Earliest visible sign of tuberous sclerosis. Arch Dermatol 1968;98:1–6.
30. Crespo-Erchiga V, Florence VD. Malessezia yeasts and pityriasis versicolor. Curr Opin Infect Dis 2006;19:139–47.
31. Faergemann J. Pityrosporum infections. J Am Acad Dermatol 1994;31:518–20.
32. Kim NY, Pandya AG. Pigmentary diseases, office dermatology Part I. Med Clin North Am 1998;82:1185–207.
33. Lebwohl MG, Heymann WR, Berth-Jones J, et al. Treatment of skin disease: comprehensive therapeutic strategies. 2nd edition. Philadelphia: Mosby Elsevier; 2006. p. 654–6.
34. Partap R, Kaur I, Chakrabart A, et al. Single dose fluconazole versus itraconazole in pityriasis versicolor. Dermatology 2004;208:55–9.

35. Kligman AM, Willis I. A new formula for depigmenting human skin. Arch Dermatol 1978;111:40–8.
36. Pathak MA, Fitzpatrick TB, Parish JA, et al. Treatment of melasma with hydroquinone. J Invest Dermatol 1981;76:324–9.
37. Perez MI. The stepwise approach to the treatment of melasma. Cutis 2005;75: 217–22.
38. Halder RM, Richards GM. Topical agents used in the management of hyperpigmentation. Skin Therapy Lett 2004;9:1–3.
39. Nanda S, Grover C, Reddy BS, et al. Efficacy of hydroquinone 2% versus tretinoin 0.025% as adjunct topical agents for chemical peeling in patients of melasma. Dermatol Surg 2004;30:385–8.
40. Grimes PE. Melasma etiologies and therapeutic considerations. Arch Dermatol 1995;131:1453–7.
41. Wang CC, Hui CY, Sue YM, et al. Intense pulsed light for the treatment of refractory melasma in Asian persons. Dermatol Surg 2004;30:1196–200.
42. Contact dermatitis and drug reactions. In: James WD, Bergen TG, Elston DM, editors. Andrews textbook of dermatology. 10th edition. Philadelphia: Saunders Elsevier; 2006.
43. Pietrangelo A. Hereditary hemachromatosis, a new look at an old disease. N Engl J Med 2004;350:2383–97.
44. Graham Brown RAC, Sarkany I. The hepatobiliary system and the skin. In: Freedberg IM, Eisen AZ, Wolff K, et al, editors. Fitzpatrick's dermatology in general medicine. New York: McGraw-Hill; 1999. p. 1918–29.
45. Stuart CA, Pate CJ, Peter EJ. Prevalence of ancanthosis nigricans in an unselected population. Am J Med 1989;87:269–72.
46. Schwartz RA. Acanthosis nigricans. J Am Acad Dermatol 1994;3:1–19.
47. Graham-Brown RAC, Rathbone B, Marks J. The skin and disorders of the alimentary tract. In: Freedberg IM, Eisen AZ, Wolff K, et al, editors. Fitzpatrick's dermatology in general medicine. 5th edition. New York: McGraw-Hill; 1999. p. 1909–18.
48. Rosenbach A, Ram R. Treatment of acanthosis nigricans of the axillae using a long pulsed (5 msec) alexandrite laser. Dermatol Surg 2004;30:1158–60.
49. Rosser T, Packer RJ. Neurofibromas in children with neurofibromatosis 1. J Child Neurol 2002;17(8):585–91.
50. Friedman JM. Neurofibromatosis 1: clinical manifestations and diagnostic criteria. J Child Neurol 2002;17(8):548–54.
51. Landau M, Kratchik BR. The diagnostic value of café au lait macules. J Am Acad Dermatol 1999;40:877–90.
52. Genodermatoses and congenital anomalies. In: James WD, Bergen TG, Elston DM, editors. Andrews textbook of dermatology. 10th edition. Philadelphia: Saunders Elsevier; 2006. p. 547–80.
53. Martuza R, Eldridge R. Neurofibromatosis 2. N Engl J Med 1988;318:684.

Malignant Skin Neoplasms

Carlos Ricotti, MD[a], Navid Bouzari, MD[b], Amar Agadi, MD[c], Clay J. Cockerell, MD[a,c],*

KEYWORDS

- Skin cancer • Basal cell carcinoma • Melanoma
- Squamous cell carcinoma • Skin neoplasms

Skin cancer is the most common form of cancer in the United States, with the incidence increasing considerably. At current rates in the United States, a skin cancer will develop in 1 in 6 people during their lifetime.[1] The most common of skin cancers may be categorized into 2 major groups: melanoma and nonmelanoma skin cancers. The latter group consists primarily of basal cell carcinomas and squamous cell carcinomas. Roughly 1,200,000 nonmelanoma skin cancers develop annually in the United States.[2] These tumors are rarely fatal, but are considered to be fast growing tumors that if neglected may be locally and functionally destructive.

In contrast, melanoma represents 5% of all diagnosed cancers in the United States, 15% of which prove to be fatal.[3] Although melanoma is seen more with increasing age, it is the most frequent cancer plaguing women aged 25 to 29 years, and the second most frequent cancer afflicting women aged 30 to 34.[2] Tumor depth is the most important prognostic indicator for melanoma, thus early recognition and management are imperative for improved therapeutic outcome.

Although the nonmelanoma and melanoma skin cancers encompass the vast majority of skin cancers, there is a large number of other malignancies of the skin that are less commonly confronted by the clinician. Neoplasms of the skin classically have been divided into those that differentiate from the epidermis, dermis, adnexal structures of the skin, and those derived systemically. This review focuses on the most frequent malignant neoplasms, and divides them into those that are classically designated nonmelanoma skin cancers (also known as keratinocytic tumors), melanoma, and other less common skin cancers of the skin. An extensive list of skin malignancies is provided in **Box 1**.

[a] Department of Dermatology, University of Texas Southwestern Medical Center, 5323 Harry Hines Boulevard, Dallas, TX 75390-9069, USA
[b] Department of Dermatology, University of Miami L. Miller School of Medicine, 1600 NW 10th Avenue, Miami, FL 33136, USA
[c] Cockerell and Associates Dermatopathology Laboratories/Dermpath Diagnostics, 2330 Butler Street Suite 115, Dallas, TX 75235, USA
* Corresponding author. Cockerell and Associates Dermatopathology Laboratories/Dermpath Diagnostics, 2330 Butler Street Suite 115, Dallas, TX 75235.
E-mail address: ccockerell@dermpathdiagnostics.com (C.J. Cockerell).

Med Clin N Am 93 (2009) 1241–1264
doi:10.1016/j.mcna.2009.08.011
0025-7125/09/$ – see front matter © 2009 Elsevier Inc. All rights reserved.

Box 1
Malignant skin neoplasms

1. Keratinocytic tumors
   a. basal cell carcinoma
   b. squamous cell carcinoma
   c. Bowen's disease
   d. bowenoid papulosis
   e. actinic keratosis
   f. keratoacanthoma
2. Melanocytic tumors
   a. superficial spreading melanoma
   b. nodular melanoma
   c. lentigo maligna
   d. acral-lentiginous melanoma
   e. desmoplastic melanoma
   f. nevoid melanoma
   g. amelanotic melanoma
3. Appendageal tumors
   a. tubular carcinoma
   b. microcystic adnexal carcinoma
   c. porocarcinoma
   d. spiradenocarcinoma
   e. hidradenocarcinoma
   f. mucinous carcinoma
   g. digital papillary carcinoma
   h. apocrine carcinoma
   i. Paget's disease and extramammary Paget's disease
4. Soft tissue tumors
   a. dermatofibrosarcoma protuberans
   b. Kaposi sarcoma
   c. angiosarcoma
5. Neural tumors
   a. primary malignant peripheral neuroectodermal tumor
   b. Merkel cell carcinoma
6. Cutaneous lymphomas

NONMELANOMA SKIN CANCERS (KERATINOCYTIC TUMORS)
Actinic Keratosis (Solar Keratosis)

Actinic keratosis was first identified as "keratoma senilis" by Freudenthal in 1926, and later more fully described and renamed "actinic keratosis" by Pinkus in 1958.[4,5] The term "actinic keratosis" literally means a keratotic (thickened, scaly) growth caused by damage induced by a ray, presumably electromagnetic irradiation including sunlight. Other sources of radiation such as artificial light sources, including tanning beds and ultraviolet irradiation, may result in actinic keratosis as well. These lesions are considered to be premalignant squamoproliferative lesions, and some investigators have postulated that they may actually represent an intraepithelial form of squamous cell carcinoma kept in check by immune surveillance of the body.

Actinic keratosis is one of the most common skin conditions managed by the dermatologist. There are more than 2 million cases diagnosed yearly. In Australia, the estimated rates of actinic keratosis in adults over 40 years old ranges from 40% to 60%.[6] It is estimated that up to 25% regress spontaneously but 0.1% to 10% may undergo malignant transformation to squamous cell carcinoma.[7–9]

The frequency of actinic keratosis correlates with cumulative UV exposure. High-risk populations include the elderly and people receiving immunosuppressive therapy, psoralen plus ultraviolet A therapy, and arsenic exposure. Outdoor workers have higher annual exposure to ultraviolet light, thus constituting an occupational risk in a subset of patients.[10–12]

In solid organ transplant patients, actinic keratosis occurs significantly earlier (54 vs 70 years).[13] Furthermore, it has been suggested that in patients with organ transplants and actinic keratosis, there is a higher accelerated progress of squamoproliferative neoplasms to invasive squamous cell carcinoma.[14]

Actinic keratosis clinically presents as rough, pink, but circumscribed epidermal lesions (<1 cm in diameter), typically found on areas of the body exposed to sunlight (**Fig. 1**); it can also present with brown pigmentation, and may form cutaneous horns (**Fig. 2**). Patients of fair complexion and chronic sun exposure most commonly have actinic keratosis, but it can occur in patients of any skin type. Due to the variety of clinical presentations, other lesions such as melanomas, squamous cell carcinomas, and warts must be excluded. It is more difficult to separate actinic keratosis from other skin neoplasms in patients with multiple actinic keratosis. Furthermore it is difficult, if not impossible, to determine which actinic keratosis will eventually become a squamous cell carcinoma.

Actinic keratoses represent focal areas of abnormal keratinocyte proliferation with loss of orderly maturation of keratinocytes. There are atypical keratinocytes characteristically involving the lower portions of the epidermis with overlying parakeratosis (**Fig. 3**). Cells show hyperchromaticity of nuclei, and atypical mitotic figures. Five classic histologic variants have been described: hypertrophic, atrophic, bowenoid, acantholytic, and pigmented. Histologic overlap of more advanced actinic keratosis and squamous cell carcinoma in situ is frequent, and some investigators have postulated a revised histologic grading system similar to that of cervical intraepithelial neoplasms (squamous cell carcinoma in situ AK type or keratinocyte intraepithelial neoplasia). Identical gene mutations (ie, p53) have been linked to both actinic keratosis and squamous cell carcinoma, supporting the hypothesis that actinic keratosis is indeed an early squamous cell carcinoma in situ.[15] This linkage would potentially allow grading of these lesions, and help improve the understanding of their biologic behavior.

Actinic keratoses may be treated for cosmetic reasons or for relief of associated symptoms, but the most compelling reason for treatment is to prevent squamous cell carcinomas. Several treatment modalities have been described including

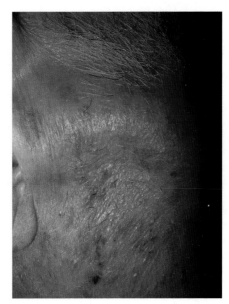

Fig. 1. Actinic keratosis. There are multiple pink scaly papules. Multiple lesions are frequently seen, and it is difficult to distinguish more advanced lesions from squamous cell carcinoma.

cryotherapy, photodynamic therapy, and topical therapies. Choice of treatment depends on patient preference and understanding of treatment, comorbidity, and cost. Whereas cryotherapy and other surgical therapies (eg, laser therapy, dermabrasion, and so forth) are suitable for treating solitary or few actinic keratosis, more widespread change requires topical treatment or photodynamic therapy (PDT). Cryotherapy using liquid nitrogen is the most common modality for treating actinic keratoses. The procedure is highly effective, with reported cure rates between 75% and 99%.[16] Potential adverse effects include infection, hypo- or hyperpigmentation, scarring, and hair loss; however, serious reactions are rare. Topical fluorouracil is an established treatment for actinic keratosis (**Fig. 4**). Fluorouracil acts by inhibiting DNA synthesis. Another topical treatment is imiquimod, which is an immunomodulator

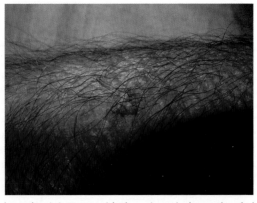

Fig. 2. A cutaneous horn (Actinic Keratosis) There is an indurated scaly horn present on the surface of a pink papule.

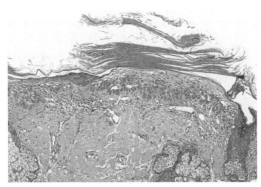

Fig. 3. Histologic image of actinic keratosis under light microscopy (original magnification ×20). There are characteristic focal areas of parakeratosis, with loss of the underlying granular layer, and a slightly thickened epidermis. There is some mild downward growth of the basal layer and cytologically atypical keratinocytes. Extensive solar elastosis is commonly observed in the dermis. If solar elastosis is not evident in a suspected actinic keratosis, other lesions that mimic actinic keratosis should be considered in the differential diagnosis.

that acts by upregulating the production of tumor necrosis factor-α and other proinflammatory cytokines in the skin via Toll-like receptors. Fluorouracil is approved in both the United States and Europe for treating actinic keratosis, with reported clearance rates between 53.7% and 70%.[17] Topical diclofenac has also been suggested to improve clinical appearance of actinic keratosis in several studies. In a phase 4 study, 78% of patients had 75% reduction in actinic keratosis after 12 weeks of treatment with topical diclofenac. However, its efficacy has not been confirmed histologically, and there is a need for further studies. Photodynamic therapy involves applying a photosensitizing agent to each actinic keratosis, followed by exposure to light of a specific wavelength; this leads to cell death. This method has been found to be superior to cryotherapy and 5-fluorouracil (5-FU) in treating extensive actinic keratosis, with a reported cure rate between 69% and 93%. PDT using both blue light and red light is approved by the Food and Drug Administration (FDA) for treating nonhyperkeratotic actinic keratosis on the face and scalp.[16]

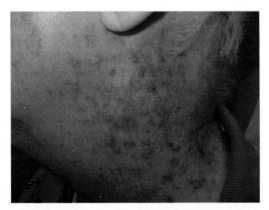

Fig. 4. Clinical presentation of a patient who received 2 weeks of topical 5-fluorouracil twice daily. There are multiple pink scaly papules and areas of erosion. Lesions resolve 1 month after therapy. Lesions that persist after therapy may represent early squamous cell carcinomas and should be managed appropriately.

Keratoacanthoma

Keratoacanthoma was first described as a "crateriform ulcer of the face" by sir Jonathan Hutchinson, and due to its considerable acanthosis was coined "keratoacanthoma" during the post-World War II era by Freudenthal of Wroclaw.[18,19]

The incidence of keratoacanthoma is difficult to know because 50% of cases spontaneously involute.[20] Data on keratoacanthoma incidence does not take this into account. Keratoacanthomas occur between the ages of 50 and 69 years, with rare presentation before the age of 20.[21,22] The incidence is slightly increased in males.[22]

The typical keratoacanthoma is a solitary lesion found on the lower lip, cheek, nose, eyelid, hands, or neck (**Fig. 5**).[23] The lesion is generally characterized by 3 distinct stages of maturation. During the primary stage the tumor grows rapidly to about 10 to 25 mm in size.[24] This stage lasts approximately 2 months. During the secondary stage the lesion stops growing and presents as a keratin-containing domelike structure. During the tertiary stage, 50% of the lesions regress and expel their keratin contents. This stage lasts approximately 1 month.[20,25] One-fifth of keratoacanthomas studied have evolved into malignant lesions metastasizing into perivascular, perineural, intravascular, and lymphatic areas.[26–28]

During the proliferative or primary stage, proximal hair follicles localize the invagination of the epidermis with a keratin inclusion. This lesion is characterized by hyperkeratosis, acanthosis, and a thick stratum granulosum with keratohyalin granules. In addition, mitotically active, possibly atypical epidermal cells migrate from the hair follicles toward the eccrine sweat glands. Perineural and intravascular invasion are considered benign, while the prognostic impact of invasion below the level of eccrine sweat glands is under debate. During the fully developed, secondary stage, a lip of epidermal cells extends around a keratin-filled crater, with many areas of keratinization characterized by an eosinophilic and glassy-finished look. Microabscesses with associated neutrophils, horn pearls, and a mixed dermal accumulation of lymphocytes, histiocytes, eosinophils, and plasma cells are common. During the involutional, or tertiary stage, keratinization of the base of the crater leads to its flattening-out. The dermal infiltrate of the secondary stage is characterized predominantly by histiocytes that form a granuloma-like structure against the keratinized base. Fibroblasts beneath the base proliferate, causing a gradual flattening of the base and expulsion of the contents of the lesion including any atypical remnants. Due to the histologic and

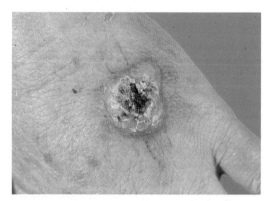

Fig. 5. A keratoacanthoma. There is a large pink plaque with raised borders and a crateriform ulcer in the center of the lesion. Crateriform squamous cell carcinomas may present clinically with similar findings.

clinical findings, many consider this a variant of squamous cell carcinoma.[24] Therapy for keratoacanthomas is primarily destruction or excision. Management is essentially similar to that of squamous cell carcinomas and basal cell carcinomas, and is discussed in a later section.

Squamous Cell Carcinoma in Situ and Bowen's Disease

Squamous cell carcinoma in situ is an "intraepidermal carcinoma" made up of atypical keratinocytes throughout the full thickness of the epidermis. Bowen's disease is a term initially historically used for squamous cell carcinoma in situ of "non–sun-exposed" skin. At present, however, it is generally accepted that Bowen's disease and squamous cell carcinoma of the skin in situ are synonymous.

The etiology of squamous cell carcinoma in situ is similar to actinic keratosis, and includes UV irradiation from sunlight or other sources. Squamous cell carcinomas are also frequently associated with human papilloma virus (HPV). Those of genital areas are most commonly associated with HPV-16 and HPV-18. Nongenital squamous cell carcinoma in situ may also be associated with HPV, those most commonly cited in the literature being HPV-2, HPV-16, HPV-34, and HPV-56. A retrospective study of patients with squamous cell carcinoma in situ showed that 19% were immunocompromised, and these patients were approximately 10 years younger, had more lesions, and had a higher rate of recurrence (9% vs 3%).[29] Roughly 3% to 11% of squamous cell carcinomas in situ may become invasive squamous cell carcinomas, and thus present invasive malignant potential.[30,31]

These lesions present clinically as pink, well-defined, erythematous papules and plaques anywhere on the body including the trunk, eyelids, hands, feet, face, and genital area. The lesions may have scale, and the patient often inform the physician that the lesion has bled in the past.

Squamous cell carcinoma in situ histologically shows full-thickness involvement of atypical keratinocytes throughout the epidermis, and may involve the epidermis of adnexal structures such as the hair follicles. Increased mitotic activity is evident, as well as disorganization of the orderly maturation of the epidermis with loss of the granular layer. Necrotic keratinocytes are frequently observed. In the superficial dermis there may be lymphocyte aggregates (**Fig. 6**).[32] Bowenoid papulosis is likely a variant of squamous cell carcinoma in situ that clinically appears on the genitals, and appears more as a verrucous simulating condyloma accuminatum (**Fig. 7**). Bowenoid papulosis histologically has features of condyloma accuminatum but also keratinocyte atypia similar to that found in squamous cell carcinoma in situ. In general these tumors are more indolent than squamous cell carcinoma in situ, but invasive bowenoid papulosis has been reported.

Multiple therapeutic options are available for treatment of squamous cell carcinoma in situ. 5-FU has been used topically for treatment of squamous cell carcinoma in situ. 5-FU is usually applied once or twice daily as a 5% cream for a variable period of time (between 1 week and 2 months) to achieve disease control, and repeated if required at intervals. Imiquimod has been used as a 5% cream. Imiquimod has both anti-HPV and antitumor effects, and is therefore potentially useful for HPV-associated Bowen/bowenoid papulosis as well as for non-HPV–associated Bowen disease. The best evidence currently available is a single small study that demonstrated 73% histologically proven resolution with imiquimod.[33] Cryotherapy seems to have a good success rate with adequate treatment (recurrences less than 10% at 12 months), but healing may be slow for broad lesions and discomfort may limit treatment of multiple lesions. Curettage with electrocautery is also described, with a wide range of cure rates. Although it is logical that excision should be an effective treatment, the evidence base is limited.

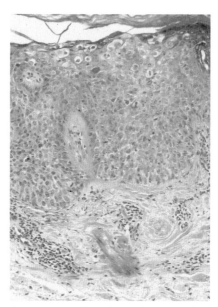

Fig. 6. Histologic image of squamous cell carcinoma in situ under light microscopy (original magnification ×20). There is full-thickness involvement of the epidermis and manifold involvement of the pilosebaceous units. There is disorderly maturation of the keratinocytes and presence of many mitoses and dyskeratotic keratinocytes throughout the epidermis. The basement membrane is not compromised, and the lesion is limited to the epidermis.

Mohs micrographic surgery (MMS) has become the recommended treatment for digital and for some cases of genital (especially penile) squamous cell carcinoma in situ, due to its tissue-sparing benefits. Previous studies on PDT suggested an initial clinical clearance rate of 80% to 100% (most around 90%) with 1 or 2 treatments, and a recurrence rate of about 0% to 10% at 12 months. This modality requires the activation of a photosensitizer, usually a porphyrin derivative, by visible light. All of the aforementioned treatments have some advantages and disadvantages, which

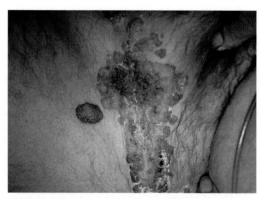

Fig. 7. Bowenoid papulosis. There is a large multifocal verrucous brown plaque with surrounding brown/red papules. These lesions tend to have irregular borders and often are confused with melanoma.

are dictated by lesional factors (size, number, site, potential for healing, or functional impairment), general health issues, availability, and cost.[34]

Squamous Cell Carcinoma

Squamous cell carcinoma is the second most common cancer in the United States, but causes more deaths than basal cell carcinoma. The American Cancer Society estimated that at least 20% of cases of skin cancer in the year 2000 were squamous cell carcinomas and in 2008, over 1 million new cases of skin cancer were estimated.[3] Squamous cell carcinoma is more common in older, fair-skinned individuals, and is a result of chronic UV exposure. The pathomechanism for the development of squamous cell carcinoma is complex and multifactorial, and requires both genetic predisposition and environmental exposures. The role of UV damage to the DNA of keratinocytes is considered the most important contributing carcinogenic factor, as 80% of squamous cell carcinomas occur on sun-exposed areas of the body. Although both UVA and UVB radiation plays a role in the formation of squamous cell carcinoma, it seems that UVB rays are the more important contributing factor. Furthermore, it is known that the incidence is increasing, and that this may due to the depleting ozone layer, further migration of aging populations to areas of warmer climate, and the increased use of tanning beds.[35] Duration of immunosuppression in solid organ transplanted patients has been directly correlated with the development of squamous cell carcinoma in this patient subset.[36–38] The incidence increased from 5% at 2 years, to 10% to 27% at 10 years, to 40% to 60% at 20 years, and it was found to be linked to the associated immunosuppression regimen. These regimens allow for the production of cytokines that promote tumor growth and proliferation.[14] HPV plays a role in the pathogenesis of squamous cell carcinoma in both immunocompetent and immunosuppressed patients. In genital squamous cell carcinoma HPV-16 or HPV-18 have been implicated, and in head and neck squamous cell carcinoma, HPV-16 is a risk factor. Chronic inflammatory conditions may also result in keratinocyte transformation to squamous cell carcinoma. These conditions include chronic venous ulcers, discoid lupus erythematosus lesions, erosive lichen planus, and lymphedema. Any changes in the clinical appearance of a chronic cutaneous inflammatory condition, especially increased induration or ulceration, should trigger the physician to consider transformation to squamous cell carcinoma and pursue further diagnostic studies including a skin biopsy.

For most fair-skinned individuals, squamous cell carcinoma will develop on skin within a preexisting area of actinic keratosis. The clinical presentation may vary from a small, pink, erythematous, scaly papule to a large, ulcerated, and indurated plaque (**Fig. 8**). If the squamous cell carcinoma is sufficient in size, patients may note pain, bleeding, or other peripheral neural symptoms reflecting perineural spread. The clinical differential diagnosis includes actinic keratosis, keratoacanthoma, basal cell carcinoma, and melanoma. The definitive diagnosis is usually rendered on pathologic evaluation of a lesional skin biopsy specimen. Squamous cell carcinomas of mucosal surfaces tend to be far more aggressive, and may present with regional lymph node involvement. A lymphatic examination is mandatory for any invasive lesion and for patients with prior invasive or high-risk squamous cell carcinomas. For larger lesions and lesions involving the mucosal surfaces, patients should be staged according to the American Joint Committee on Cancer criteria.

Squamous cell carcinomas consist histologically of nests of atypical squamous epithelial cells intermixed with normal squamous cells, which arise from the epidermis and extend into the dermis. Characteristics of these atypical cells include a more extensive range of size and shape, hyperplasia and hyperchromasia of nuclei,

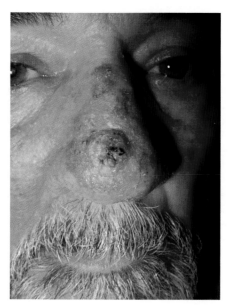

Fig. 8. An invasive squamous cell carcinoma. There is a large crusted plaque with surrounding ill-defined pink scaly plaque.

increased abnormal mitotic figures, and loss of intercellular bridges. Keratinization is common in squamous cell carcinomas (**Fig. 9**). Most squamous cell carcinomas arise at a site with surrounding chronic sun damage, showing solar elastosis as well as actinic keratosis adjacent or within the squamous cell carcinomas. Some investigators have proposed histologic criteria for determining prognosis, but currently there are no definitive criteria. Many have suggested that prognosis be based on histologic squamous cell carcinoma variant, depth of invasion, or whether there is perineural

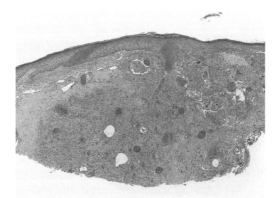

Fig. 9. Histologic image of an invasive squamous cell carcinoma under light microscopy (original magnification ×10). There is a large nest of squamous epithelial cells that arises from the epidermis and extends deep into the dermis. Cells are cytologically atypical, are large, and present with many mitotic figures. There is keratinization and squamous pearls in this lesion.

involvement, but this has yet to be generally accepted.[39] Therapy and management of squamous cell carcinomas is discussed later.

Basal Cell Carcinoma

In 1827 Arthur Jacob published "Observations respecting an ulcer of a peculiar character which affects the eyes and face."[40] What he described in his article later came to be known as basal cell carcinoma, so named because from a histologic perspective it looks similar to basal cells of the epidermis. Basal cell carcinoma is the most common malignancy occurring in humans. The American Cancer Society estimated about 75% of cases of skin cancer in the year 2000 were basal cell carcinomas and in 2008, over 1 million new cases of skin cancer were estimated.[3] Basal cell carcinoma is most common in fair-skinned individuals (those who burn easily and tan poorly), although it may be found in patients with darker skin types, including those of African descent.[41] Previous articles have suggested that childhood exposure to UV radiation is the primary cause of basal cell carcinoma, and adult exposure does not have as much of an impact.[42] Intermittent chronic light exposure, rather than continuous light exposure, is more closely associated with basal cell carcinoma.[43] The probable range of wavelength of UV exposure that contributes to all nonmelanoma skin cancers includes 293, 354, and 380 nm.[44] There is also a strong inverse correlation between latitude and the development of basal cell cancer.[45] More recently 2 vitamin D polymorphisms have been associated with nonmelanoma skin cancers and malignant melanoma, suggesting that their development may be somehow associated with vitamin D metabolism.[46] As with squamous cell cancer, basal cell carcinoma incidence increases in patients with solid organ transplantation receiving concomitant immunosuppressive therapy.[36–38]

Most basal cell carcinomas are found on the head and neck; however, some may be found in non–sun-exposed areas of the body. The vast majority (60%) of basal cell carcinomas are noduloulcerative or "rodent ulcers." These lesions begin as small, reddish, translucent nodules with telangiectasias (**Fig. 10**). As the lesion grows, the center may ulcerate, leaving behind the classic "rolled borders." If the lesion is not treated in its earlier stages it can lead to destruction of underlying tissue, including intracranial invasion.[47] Although the cancer is not known to be associated with a high mortality, there have been a few cases of metastasis to the central nervous system and the bone.[48] These cases are extremely rare, and it is much more common for basal cell carcinomas to be locally aggressive than systemically involved.

Most variants of basal cell carcinomas retain some characteristics of normal basal cells; however, they differ due to a lower cytoplasm to nuclear ratio and absence of intercellular bridges (**Fig. 11**). Different basal cell carcinomas vary in terms of change in cellular population and cell morphology. It is currently assumed that pluripotential stem cells have a high potential to convert to basal cell carcinoma when exposed to excessive sunlight or have p53 gene mutations. Four major subclasses exist: nodular, superficial, pigmented, and morpheaform. The nodular form shows palisading of nuclei, clefts between epithelium and the stroma, and a specialized stroma. The superficial form shows horizontally arranged lobules of atypical basal cells in the papillary dermis that have broad-based connections with the epidermis, surrounded by a thin stroma filled with lymphocytes and histiocytes. The pigmented form is similar to the nodular form, with the addition of melanocytes intermixed with basal cells and melanin within the cancer cells and stromal macrophages. The morpheic form has no connection to the epidermis, and usually presents as islands of neoplastic basal cells surrounded by a dense collagen-filled stroma.[49] The latter variant has

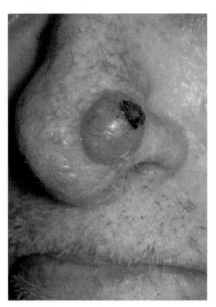

Fig. 10. A nodular basal cell carcinoma. There is a large nodule with telangiectasis and "pearly" appearance. The lesion is centrally ulcerated. Amelanotic melanoma and Merkel cell carcinoma may have similar clinical appearance.

a higher associated recurrence rate after surgical therapy compared with other variants.

The clinician should be particularly aware of patients with certain syndromes who are more predisposed to developing basal cell carcinoma frequently on non–sun-exposed skin. Xeroderma pigmentosum, an autosomal recessive condition in which repair mechanisms for UV-damaged genes are inhibited, is associated with a 1000-fold

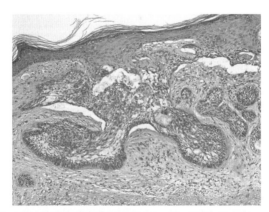

Fig. 11. Histologic image of a basal cell carcinoma under light microscopy (original magnification ×20). There are islands of basaloid cells, with palisading of the cells at the periphery and disorganized arrangement of cells within the tumor. The basaloid islands typically arise from the epidermis. Frequent histologic findings observed in this lesion are clefting of the tumor from the surrounding stroma and increased mitotic rate of cells within the tumor.

increase in skin and eye cancers, many of which are basal cell carcinomas.[50] Gorlin syndrome, also known as nevoid basal cell carcinoma syndrome, is a hereditary condition characterized by odontogenic keratocysts of the jaws, hyperkeratosis of palms and soles, and skeletal abnormalities. It was determined recently that the "Hedge Hog" pathway, including a PTCH gene mutation (this gene is involved in inhibition of a cascade molecular event that results in cell proliferation), is involved in the development of basal cell carcinomas, and this gene mutation is implicated in the pathogenesis of Gorlin syndrome. Other syndromes associated with melanin deficiency such as Rasmussen, Rombo, and albinism are associated with an increased risk of basal cell carcinoma as well.[51]

Treatment of Basal Cell Carcinoma and Squamous Cell Carcinoma

The most frequently used method for the treatment of nonmelanoma skin cancer is surgical excision of the tumor. Surgical approaches include conventional excision, MMS, electrodessication and curettage, and cryosurgery. MMS is considered by some as the "gold standard" for the treatment of a range of nonmelanoma squamous cell cancers because this method provides the most complete histologic analysis of tumor margins, the highest cure rate, and preservation of the maximal amount of normal tissue by removing the tumor with the smallest margin necessary.[52] MMS is a technique in which serial horizontal sections of tumor are removed, mapped, processed by frozen section in an en-face fashion, and analyzed microscopically. The entire deep and peripheral margins are examined by the surgeon and immediate reexcision of the residual tumor region is performed until the area is tumor free. **Table 1** shows the indications of MMS in treating nonmelanoma skin cancer. Excision is the most common therapy for treating nonmelanoma squamous cell cancer, and is useful for treating low-risk tumors because it provides acceptable cure rates and is cost-effective.[53] This method allows for histopathologic examination of the tissue, and although 100% of the margin is not examined, 95% of low-risk tumors will be adequately excised by removal of the tumor with a 4-mm margin. The cure rates for squamous cell carcinoma and basal cell cancer are 92% and 95%, respectively. Curettage and electrodessication is often used to treat superficial nonmelanoma squamous cell cancer, and relies on the textural differences between tumor cells and the surrounding normal tissue. This technique does not permit histologic margin analysis. The method is also technique dependent and not appropriate for higher-risk tumors such as morpheaform, but it is cost-effective and rapid to perform. Curettage and electrodessication is not suitable for treating recurrent tumors, lesions larger than 2 cm in diameter, tumors extending into the fat, tumors at sites of high risk for

Table 1	
Indications of Mohs micrographic surgery	
Indicated	**Preferred**
Tumor in locations with high rates of recurrence (eg, midface and ears)	Tumor in functionally and cosmetically unique areas such as the nose, lips, and eyelids
Tumors with aggressive histologic growth patterns (eg, morpheaform, infiltrative, and sclerosing BCC)	Tumor in lower extremities where healing can be prolonged and tissue preservation is advantageous
Recurrent tumor	
Tumor greater than 2 cm in size	
Tumors with ill-defined clinical margins	

recurrence, or lesions with ill-defined borders. Curettage and electrodessication has a recurrence rate of 4.5% to 17.6%.[52] Nonmelanoma squamous cell cancer can be treated using ionizing radiation as either a primary or adjuvant therapy. Although radiation therapy is effective, its use is limited because of the side effects induced; hence, radiation therapy can be used in certain patients who are not surgical candidates. Newer noninvasive options for nonmelanoma squamous cell cancer include topical chemotherapeutics, biological immune response modifiers, retinoids, and photodynamic therapy, which can be used particularly in patients with superficial tumors. Topical 5-FU application has been limited to treating superficial or squamous cell carcinoma. Topical imiquimod similarly is only effective against superficial basal cell carcinoma, small nodular basal cell carcinoma, and squamous cell carcinoma in situ. Imiquimod is FDA-approved only for actinic keratosis and superficial basal cell carcinoma. Studies have demonstrated that application of imiquimod 5 days per week for 6 weeks results in 88% histologic clearance rate using Aldara (imiquimod) 5% cream.[54] Photodynamic therapy is effective in treating squamous cell carcinoma in situ and superficial basal cell carcinomas. Photodynamic treatment of nodular basal cell carcinoma has demonstrated complete responses in 90% of patients, with 74% remaining clear after 2 years.[55] Photodynamic therapy is limited by the depth of penetration of the topical photosensitizers and should not be used to treat thick tumors, tumors with certain aggressive histologic subtypes (eg, morpheaform basal cell carcinoma), or recurrent cancers. Systemic retinoids that are derivatives of vitamin A have a proven chemopreventative effect in reducing the risk of developing squamous cell carcinoma and basal cell carcinoma. The mechanism of action is thought to occur via induction of apoptosis, impedance of tumor proliferation, or stimulation of differentiation during the tumor promotion phase of carcinogenesis. These agents, however, are typically not effective in treating existing tumors.[56]

MELANOMA
Malignant Melanoma

The American Cancer Society estimated over 62,000 newly diagnosed cases of melanoma in 2008.[3] Cutaneous melanoma may have myriad clinical appearances with histopathological correlates. Whereas most early lesions demonstrate the "ABCDEs" (Asymmetry, Borders, Color, Diameter, and Evolving) that have been described, many others may be unusual and manifest either some or none of these features. Most are patches, plaques, nodules or tumors, and are greater than 6 mm in diameter when diagnosed, but lesions much smaller than this are well recognized.

The risk factors associated with the development of malignant melanoma are also multifactorial, with both genetic and environmental factors playing a role in its pathogenesis. As with the nonmelanoma skin cancers, patients with fair skin color, blond or red hair, and who burn easily are more at risk than other patients. Details go beyond the scope of this review, but repeated acute sun exposure that has resulted in blistering sunburns during childhood or adolescence increases the risk for melanoma.[57] The effect of chronic sun exposure is more controversial, and there are conflicting data regarding the association between long-term chronic sun exposure and melanoma development.[58] The effects of UV radiation on melanocyte mutations is less understood than that of nonmelanoma skin cancers. More recently, tanning salons have been implicated in the development of malignant melanoma, and public education should be paramount in decreasing the incidence of melanoma in patients who use tanning beds.[59,60]

Malignant melanoma has been classified based on clinicopathological characteristics. The most common is the superficial spreading melanoma, followed by lentigo maligna (LM) melanoma, nodular melanoma, acral lentiginous melanoma (**Fig. 12**), desmoplastic melanoma, and other miscellaneous variants. LM and superficial spreading melanoma are both in situ melanomas, and are histologic variants of melanoma confined to the epidermis and the epidermis of adnexal structures. The other variants contain dermal components of the melanoma and, as a result, worse prognosis.

Although most malignant melanomas are pigmented, less than 2% of melanomas are amelanotic, and these pose the most difficulty in clinical diagnosis.[61] These lesions are pink or skin-colored patches, plaques, or nodules that may be ulcerated; they are often mistaken for pyogenic granuloma, basal cell carcinoma, nevi, or fibromas. Desmoplastic melanoma is a rare variant that is notoriously difficult to diagnose clinically and histologically (**Fig. 13**). Desmoplastic melanoma usually presents subtly as a pigmented or skin-colored indurated patch, papule, or plaque on sun-exposed skin. Lesions are described clinically as "fibroma" or "scar."

The histopathological diagnosis of melanoma has an extensive and detailed history. A "unifying concept" regarding the histologic diagnosis of melanoma by Ackerman has been proposed and used by the vast majority of pathologists.[62] Both architectural and cytologic criteria were established, and from these criteria the diagnosis of melanoma was rendered. The definitive diagnosis of melanoma often cannot be made, as all histologic criteria have not been fulfilled. This area of more "atypical melanocytic lesions" that do not fulfill criteria for melanoma is an ongoing area of research and investigation, and highlights the difficulty in diagnosing certain melanocytic lesions.[63]

It cannot be stressed enough that the diagnosis rendered by pathologic examination and the prognosis is dependent on appropriate and adequate sampling by the clinician.[64] Diagnosis is dependent on sampling the correct area of the lesion (ideally the whole pigmented lesion should be sampled) and examination of the entire breadth of the lesion. The lesion thickness as established by light microscopic examination is the most important determinant of prognosis, thus if the biopsy is transected at the base of the tumor, prognosis cannot be fully determined. Extent of anatomic tumor invasion by the primary lesion predicts the 10-year survival probability (**Table 2**).[65] Furthermore, this information is used to establish staging according to the American Joint Committee on Cancer Staging System.[66] Once the lesion is greater than 1 mm in depth, it has been determined that histologic observation of ulceration is a significant

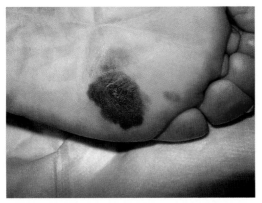

Fig. 12. An acral melanoma. There is a large (>6 mm), asymmetric, ill-defined brown patch on the sole of the patient's foot. This appearance is characteristic of advanced acral melanomas.

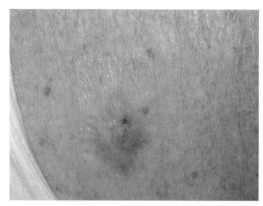

Fig. 13. A desmoplastic melanoma. The lesion is a pink, erythematous, ill-defined plaque that has a central ulcer. These lesions are frequently misdiagnosed clinically as superficial basal cell carcinomas.

prognostic indicator,[67] likely due to the related aggressiveness of the tumor or delayed diagnosis of the lesion. Other factors implicated in the prognosis of melanoma include melanoma invasion of lymphatics, angioinvasion, perineural invasion, melanoma nest satellites distal to the primary tumor, elevated lactate dehydrogenase levels, anatomic location (head and neck lesions with worse prognosis), and increased mitotic rate.

The diagnosis of melanoma can be difficult and more recently, molecular diagnostic methods, such as using comparative genomic hybridization, have allowed the measurement of copy number gene aberrations in tumors. It was discovered that over 95% of melanomas have chromosomal abnormalities whereas the majority of benign nevi do not.[68] Distinct patterns of genetic alterations, both chromosomal aberrations and the frequency of specific gene mutations, suggest that the various subtypes of melanoma arise from separate mechanistic routes in response to different selective influences.[69] For example, a study looking at the genetic alterations of melanoma found that those melanomas on skin without chronic sun-induced damage had frequent losses of chromosome 10 and frequent mutations in BRAF, whereas melanomas on skin with chronic sun-induced damage had frequent increases in the number of copies of the CCND1 gene and infrequent mutations in BRAF. KIT has also been identified as an oncogene and potential therapeutic target in melanomas of mucosal membranes, acral skin, and skin with chronic sun-induced damage. This finding is of value, as this subset of melanomas infrequently shows mutations in BRAF.[70] The observation of such chromosomal aberrations in melanoma, and a virtual

Table 2		
Melanoma prognosis based on Clark level		
Clark Level	**Histologic Location of Melanoma Cells**	**10-Year Survival**
Level I	Epidermis	99%
Level II	Penetrating the papillary dermis	96%
Level III	Filling the papillary dermis	90%
Level IV	Extending to the reticular dermis	67%
Level V	Invasion of the subcutis	26%

deficiency of abnormalities in benign nevi, leads to the possibility that chromosomal analysis could be used diagnostically in melanocytic lesions that are ambiguous, based on current methods of assessment.

Melanoma Therapy

Surgical excision is the standard of care for all primary melanomas, and consists of en bloc excision of the tumor or biopsy site with a margin containing normal appearing skin and underlying subcutaneous tissue. For decades, excision margins of 5 cm or greater in all directions from the tumor border were the standard of care. However, a recent meta-analysis showed no statistically significant difference in overall mortality when comparing wide versus narrow excision margins. Based on the World Health Organization, Australian, and European trials, a 1-cm margin is accepted as adequate for thin melanomas. The recommended maximum margin for melanomas between 1 and 4 mm is 2 cm.[71] Controversy exists around the significance of the early detection and management of microscopically positive lymph nodes detected by sentinel lymph node biopsy. Nonetheless, complete lymphadenectomy is recommended when positive nodes are detected.[72] Metastatic disease is incurable in most affected people, because melanoma does not respond to most systemic treatments. A recent Cochrane review showed an increased response to treatment when immunotherapy was added to chemotherapy, but no difference was seen in survival rate and toxic effects were increased.[73]

The outcome of melanoma depends on the stage at presentation. LM is by definition a Stage 0 disease; it is a malignancy in situ. LM has not ventured beyond the basement membrane into the dermis where lymphovascular invasion and subsequent metastases become possible. Therefore, it is curable if completely excised. Controversy exists regarding the surgical margins. Despite the general agreement of 5-mm surgical margin, it is shown to be adequate in less than 50% of cases of LM.[74] MMS offers intraoperative margin assessment, but its drawback lies in the interpretation of frozen sectioned melanocytic lesions. When surgery is technically difficult or cosmetically undesired, other methods can be employed such as cryotherapy, laser therapy, radiation therapy, and immunotherapy (eg, imiquimod). The challenge is to strike a balance between the risks and benefits of a given therapeutic approach.[75]

OTHER MALIGNANT CUTANEOUS NEOPLASMS
Merkel Cell Carcinoma

Merkel cell carcinoma, otherwise known as primary cutaneous neuroendocrine carcinoma, was initially described as trabecular carcinoma by Toker in 1972.[76] Merkel cell carcinoma became the official name due to the presence of neuroendocrine granules within the cells, which is a characteristic feature of Merkel cells.[77]

The age-adjusted incidence of Merkel cell carcinoma is 0.24 in 100,000 person-years. The incidence is higher in men than women, and it is considered primarily a disease of older or immunosuppressed Caucasian individuals. The incidence in one study in those 65 to 74 years old was 15 times that of those younger than 65.[78] Because the lesion appears most frequently on the head and neck, UV radiation is thought to be a major factor that contributes to its development. Because these lesions may appear on non–sun-exposed areas (though less frequently), genetics is thought to play a role as well. Recently the Merkel cell polyomavirus has been cited as a contributing factor to the development of Merkel cell carcinoma.[79]

The classic presentation of a Merkel cell carcinoma is a single, smooth, violet nodule on solar-damaged skin near the periorbital area with telangiectasias found overlying the nodule (**Fig. 14**). When it begins growing, it starts slowly but then progresses to more rapid growth, which usually portends a poor prognosis. Eleven to fifteen percent of patients have positive nodes on presentation, and 50% have metastasis to regional lymph nodes. Fifty percent have distant metastasis to distant nodes, liver, bone, brain, lung, and skin.[78]

The tumor is comprised histologically of small, round to oval cells of uniform size, with a vesicular nucleus and multiple small nucleoli (**Fig. 15**). Mitoses and apoptotic bodies are frequently observed. The tumor can mimic histologically both basal cell carcinoma and small cell carcinomas of the lung. Merkel cell carcinomas characteristically stain positively with CK20 and neuron-specific enolase, differentiating it from other primary tumors of the skin such as basal cell carcinoma. It has recently been reported that tumor depth on histologic evaluation may be a factor in the prognosis of these patients.[80]

Surgery is the mainstay of treatment, with guidelines recommending MMS over conventional surgery, and wide local excision of the primary site with all efforts focused on the achievement of clear surgical margins during initial resection. Guidelines recommend sentinel lymph node biopsy to maximize the detection and care of regional disease. Based on the stage of the disease, adjuvant therapies such as radiotherapy and chemotherapy may be indicated. The addition of postsurgical locoregional radiotherapy tends to decrease local and regional recurrence rates, and to prolong relapse-free survival. However, the role of chemotherapy in the treatment of Merkel cell carcinoma remains controversial.[81]

Microcystic Adnexal Carcinoma

Microcystic adnexal carcinomas are rare, aggressive tumors that were first documented in 1982. The median age of patients with these carcinomas is 56 years, with approximately equal sex distribution. Microcystic adnexal carcinoma has primarily been documented to affect whites; however, there has been one case reported in a black patient.

Case reports primarily describe a pale yellow nodule or plaque with irregular borders, which may take decades to reach full symptomatic potential. Common areas of distribution include the nasolabial and periorbital areas in the majority, with some

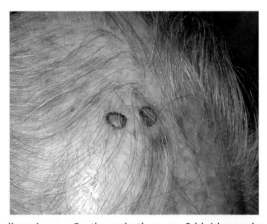

Fig. 14. A Merkel cell carcinoma. On the scalp there are 2 bluish papules that have telangiectasis. The clinician submitted the lesion as a basal cell carcinoma. The biopsy (**Fig. 15**) proved it to be a Merkel cell carcinoma.

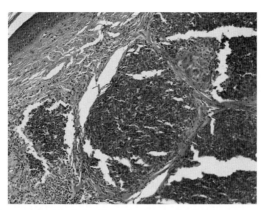

Fig. 15. Histologic image of a Merkel cell carcinoma under light microscopy (original magnification ×20). On low magnification these tumors mimic basal cell carcinomas. The tumors do not show clefting or mucin typically seen in basal cell carcinomas. There are round, small, oval cells uniform in size with multiple nucleoli. Mitosis and apoptotic figures are numerous. The cells are present in sheets and nests, infiltrating deep into the dermis. Merkel cell carcinomas show a characteristic perinuclear dot pattern, with CK20 immunoperoxidase staining assisting in the diagnosis.

rare cases demonstrating lesions in the axilla, buttocks, or scalp. The disease is known to be locally aggressive, with cases where it has invaded as deeply as skeletal muscle. There have been only a few cases of metastasis.[82–84]

The lesion originates in the dermis and is poorly circumscribed. Basaloid keratinocytes and ducts are 2 primary components. The keratinocyte component may have horn cysts and premature hair follicles. As the cancer extends through the dermis to deeper layers, the keratinocyte/ductal islands reduce in size.[52]

Mucinous Carcinoma

Mucinous carcinoma is thought to arise from sweat glands. It is estimated that the annual incidence of mucinous carcinoma is 0.1 per million.[85] This figure may be underestimated because mucinous carcinoma is often mistaken for a benign tumor.

The tumor clinically presents as a skin-colored to bluish subcutaneous or superficial lesion, most often located in the area of the eyelid. This lesion can be primary or secondary to an underlying malignancy. Internal malignancies of the colon and breast must be ruled out by the clinician, based on clinical, radiologic, and pathologic correlation.

The tumor is composed histopathologically of groups of epithelial cells in the form of ducts, nests, or cords, which are separated by clear areas that contain cells containing mucin. The epithelial cells are strongly positive for periodic acid Schiff and Alcian blue at a pH of 2.5.[52]

Management includes full workup to exclude the possibility of underlying malignancy, and to determine if the lesion is primary excision with appropriate margins. MMS has been previously used to cure primary lesions.[86]

Aggressive Digital Papillary Adenocarcinoma

Just as with the other sweat gland carcinomas mentioned (microcystic adnexal carcinoma and mucinous carcinoma), this is a rare condition. Most cases have been in men in their sixth and eighth decades, although there have been a few in individuals younger than 20 years.

On presentation, lesions may be painful and mimic a benign "cyst," pyogenic granuloma, soft tissue infection, or a nonspecific ulcer. Thus, aggressive adenocarcinoma of the digit should be suspected clinically in a patient with a painful tumor of the digit.[87]

This tumor is marked by dermal ductal and tubuloalveolar structures, which have papilla that project into cystlike openings. In addition, these papilla are lined by epithelial cells that project into smaller cystlike structures. Recurrence rates without appropriate excision approach 50%, but surgical reexcision or amputation with negative histologic margins reduce recurrence rates to 5%.[88]

SUMMARY

Skin cancers may be derived from any part of the skin, and the classification of all variants is extensive. Overall they are the most common cancers of the body, and include those that are highly mortal and those that are associated with an increased morbidity. In this review the most common skin cancers confronted by the clinician and their management are discussed. New associations are highlighted, as well as new information that can help the clinician to better understand the pathogenesis of many of these entities.

REFERENCES

1. Gloster HM, Brodland DG. The epidemiology of skin cancer. Dermatol Surg 1996; 22:217–26.
2. Miller DL, Weinstock MA. Nonmelanoma skin cancer in the United States: incidence. J Am Acad Dermatol 1994;30:774–8.
3. American Cancer Society, 2008 statistics. Available at: http://www.cancer.org/downloads/STT/2008CAFFfinalsecured.pdf. Accessed June 10, 2009.
4. Freudenthal W. Verruca senilis und Keratoma senile. Arch Dermatol Syphilol (Berlin) 1926;158:539–44 [in German].
5. Pinkus H. Keratosis senilis: a biologic concept of its pathogenesis and diagnosis based on the study of normal epidermis and 1730 seborrheic and senile keratoses. Am J Clin Pathol 1958;29:193–207.
6. Green A, Beardmore G, Hart V, et al. Skin cancer in a Queensland population. J Am Acad Dermatol 1988;19:1045–52.
7. Marks R, Foley P, Goodman G, et al. Spontaneous remission of solar keratoses: the case for conservative management. Br J Dermatol 1986;155:649–55.
8. Marks R, Rennie G, Selwood TS. Malignant transformation of solar keratoses to squamous cell carcinoma. Lancet 1988;1:795–7.
9. Dodson JM, DeSpain J, Hewett JE, et al. Malignant potential of actinic keratoses and the controversy over treatment. Arch Dermatol 1991;127:1029–31.
10. Chuang TY, Heinreich LA, Shultz MD, et al. PUVA and skin cancer, a historical cohort study on 492 patients. J Am Acad Dermatol 1992;26(2 Pt 1):173–7.
11. Beirn SF, Judge P, Urbach F, et al. Skin cancer in County Galway, Ireland. Proc Natl Cancer Conf 1970;6:489–500.
12. Schwartz RA. Premalignant keratinocytic neoplasms. J Am Acad Dermatol 1996; 35:223–42.
13. Boyd AS, Stasko T, Cameron GS, et al. Histologic features of actinic keratosis in solid organ transplant recipients and healthy controls. J Am Acad Dermatol 2001; 45:217–21.

14. Guba M, Graeb C, Jauch KW, et al. Pro- and anti-cancer effects of immunosuppressive agents used in organ transplantation. Transplantation 2004;77:1777–82.
15. Fu W, Cockerell C. The actinic (solar) keratosis: a 21st-century perspective. Arch Dermatol 2003;139:66–70.
16. McIntyre WJ, Downs M, Bedwell SA. Treatment options for actinic keratosis. Am Fam Physician 2007;76(5):667–71.
17. Vatve M, Ortonne JP, Birch-Machin MA, et al. Management of field change in actinic keratosis. Br J Dermatol 2007;157(Suppl 2):21–4.
18. Hutchinson JA. Morbid growths and tumours: the crateriform ulcer of the face, a form of acute epithelial cancer. Trans Pathol Soc Lond 1889;40:275–81.
19. Rudolph R, Gray AP, Leipold HW. Intracutaneous cornifying epithelioma ("keratoacanthoma") of dogs and keratoacanthoma of man. Cornell Vet 1977;67:254–64.
20. Griffiths RW. Keratoacanthoma observed. Br J Plast Surg 2004;57:485–501.
21. Schwartz RA. Keratoacanthoma: a clinico-pathologic enigma. Dermatol Surg 2004;30:326–33.
22. Buescher L, DeSpain JD, Diaz-Arias AA, et al. Keratoacanthoma arising in an organoid nevus during childhood: case report and literature review. Pediatr Dermatol 1991;8:117–9.
23. Oh CK, Son HS, Lee JB, et al. Intralesional interferon alfa-2b treatment of keratoacanthomas. J Am Acad Dermatol 2004;51:S177–80.
24. Kwittken J. A histologic chronology of the clinical course of the keratocarcinoma (so called keratoacanthoma). Mt Sinai J Med 1975;42:127–35.
25. Seifert A, Nasemann T. Keratoacanthoma and its clinical variants. Review of the literature and histopathologic analysis of 90 cases. Hautarzt 1989;40:189–202.
26. Beham A, Regauer S, Soyer HP, et al. Keratoacanthoma: a clinically distinct variant of well differentiated squamous cell carcinoma. Adv Anat Pathol 1998;5:269–80.
27. Batinac T, Zamolo G, Coklo M, et al. Possible key role of granzyme B in keratoacanthoma regression. Med Hypotheses 2006;66:1129–32.
28. Gottfarstein-Maruani A, Michenet P, Kerdraon R, et al. Keratoacanthoma: two cases with intravascular spread. Ann Pathol 2003;23:438–42.
29. Drake AL, Walling HW. Variations in presentation of squamous cell carcinoma in situ (Bowen's disease) in immunocompromised patients. J Am Acad Dermatol 2008;59(1):68–71.
30. Kao GF. Carcinoma arising in Bowen's disease. Arch Dermatol 1986;122:1124.
31. Graham JH, Helwig EB. Bowen's disease and its relationship to systemic cancer. Arch Dermatol 1959;80:133.
32. Lee MM, Wick MM. Bowen's disease. Clin Dermatol 1993;11:43–6.
33. Patel GK, Goodwin R, Chawla M, et al. Imiquimod 5% cream monotherapy for cutaneous squamous cell carcinoma in situ (Bowen's disease): a randomised, double-blind, placebo-controlled trial. J Am Acad Dermatol 2006;54:1025–32.
34. Cox NH, Eedy DJ, Morton CA, et al. British Association of Dermatologists. Guidelines for management of Bowen's disease: 2006 update. Br J Dermatol 2007;156(1):11–21.
35. Karagas MR, Stannard VA, Mott LA, et al. Use of tanning devices and risk of basal cell and squamous cell skin cancers. J Natl Cancer Inst 2002;94(3):224–6.
36. Kasiske BL, Snyder JJ, Gilbertson DT, et al. Cancer after kidney transplantation in the United States. Am J Transplant 2004;4:905–13.
37. Ramsay HM, Reece SM, Fryere AA, et al. Seven-year prospective study of non-melanoma skin cancer incidence in UK renal transplant recipients. Transplantation 2007;84:437–9.

38. Bordea C, Wojnarowska F, Millard PR, et al. Skin cancers in renal-transplant recipients occur more frequently than previously recognized in a temperate climate. Transplantation 2004;77:574–9.

39. Cassarino DS, Derienzo DP, Barr RJ. Cutaneous squamous cell carcinoma: a comprehensive clinicopathologic classification—part two. J Cutan Pathol 2006;33(4):261–79.

40. Crouch HE. History of basal cell carcinoma and its treatment. J R Soc Med 1983; 76(4):302–6.

41. Nouri K, Romanelli P, Trent J, et al. Rare presentation of basal cell carcinoma. J Cutan Med Surg 2002;6(3):226–8.

42. Kricker A, Armstrong B, English D, et al. A case-control study of non-melanocytic skin cancer and sun exposure in Western Australia. J Cancer Res Clin Oncol 1991;117(Suppl II):S75.

43. Kricker A, Armstrong BK, English DR, et al. Does intermittent sun exposure cause basal cell carcinoma? a case-control study in Western Australia. Int J Cancer 1995;60:489–94.

44. De Gruijl FR, Sterenborg HJ, Forbes PD, et al. Wavelength dependence of skin cancer induction by ultraviolet irradiation of albino hairless mice. Cancer Res 1993;52:1–8.

45. Scotto J, Fears TR, Fraumeni JF. Incidence of nonmelanoma skin cancer in the United States. Washington, DC: US Department of Health and Human Services; 1983.

46. Gandini S, Raimondi S, Gnagnarella P, et al. Vitamin D and skin cancer: a meta-analysis. Eur J Cancer 2009;45(4):634–41 [Epub 2008 Nov 12].

47. Kleydman Y, Manolidis S, Ratner D. Basal cell cancer with intracranial invasion. J Am Acad Dermatol 2009;60(6):1045–9.

48. Elghissassi I, Mikou A, Inrhaoun H, et al. Metastatic basal cell carcinoma to the bone and bone marrow. Int J Dermatol 2009;48(5):481–3.

49. Elder D, Elenitsas R, Johnson B Jr, et al, editors. Lever's histopathology of the skin. 9th edition. Philadelphia: Lippincott Williams and Wilkins; 2005. p. 715–1157.

50. Kraemer KH, Lee MM, Scotto J. Xeroderma pigmentosum: cutaneous, ocular, and neurologic abnormalities in 830 published cases. Arch Dermatol 1987;123: 241–50.

51. Xie J, Murone M, Luoh SM, et al. Activating smoothened mutations in sporadic basal-cell carcinoma. Nature 1998;391:90–2.

52. Neville JA, Welch E, Leffell DJ. Management of nonmelanoma skin cancer in 2007. Nat Clin Pract Oncol 2007;4(8):462–9.

53. Nguyen T, Ho D. Nonmelanoma skin cancer. Curr Treat Options Oncol 2002;3: 193–203.

54. Available at: http://www.fda.gov/cder/foi/label/2004/20723s016lbl.pdf. Accessed August 1, 2009.

55. Rhodes LE. Photodynamic therapy using topical methyl aminolevulinate vs. surgery for nodular basal cell carcinoma. Arch Dermatol 2004;4:17–23.

56. Kovach BT, Murphy G, Otley CC, et al. Oral retinoids for chemoprevention of skin cancers in organ transplant recipients: results of a survey. Transplant Proc 2006; 38(5):1366–8.

57. Beral V, Evans S, Shaw H, et al. Cutaneous factors related to the risk of malignant melanoma. Br J Dermatol 1983;109(2):165–72.

58. Pfahlberg A, Kölmel KF, Gefeller O, Febim Study Group. Timing of excessive ultraviolet radiation and melanoma: epidemiology does not support the existence

of a critical period of high susceptibility to solar ultraviolet radiation-induced melanoma. Br J Dermatol 2001;144(3):471–5.

59. Clough-Gorr KM, Titus-Ernstoff L, Perry AE, et al. Exposure to sunlamps, tanning beds, and melanoma risk. Cancer Causes Control 2008;19(7):659–69.

60. Ting W, Schultz K, Cac NN, et al. Tanning bed exposure increases the risk of malignant melanoma. Int J Dermatol 2007;46(12):1253–7.

61. Giuliano AE, Cochran AJ, Morton DL. Melanoma from unknown primary site and amelanotic melanoma. Semin Oncol 1982;9(4):442–7.

62. Ackerman AB. Malignant melanoma. A unifying concept. Am J Dermatopathol 1980;2(4):309–13.

63. Ludgate MW, Fullen DR, Lee J, et al. The atypical Spitz tumor of uncertain biologic potential: a series of 67 patients from a single institution. Cancer 2009; 115(3):631–41.

64. Tran KT, Wright NA, Cockerell CJ. Biopsy of the pigmented lesion—when and how. J Am Acad Dermatol 2008;59(5):852–71.

65. Clark WH Jr, From L, Bernardino EA, et al. The histogenesis and biologic behavior of primary human malignant melanomas of the skin. Cancer Res 1969;29(3): 705–27.

66. Balch CM, Buzaid AC, Soong SJ, et al. Final version of the American Joint Committee on Cancer staging system for cutaneous melanoma. J Clin Oncol 2001;19(16):3635–48.

67. Balch CM, Wilkerson JA, Murad TM, et al. The prognostic significance of ulceration of cutaneous melanoma. Cancer 1980;45(12):3012–7.

68. Bastian BC. Molecular genetics of melanocytic neoplasia: practical applications for diagnosis. Pathology 2004;36(5):458–61.

69. Curtin JA, Fridlyand J, Kageshita T, et al. Distinct sets of genetic alterations in melanoma. N Engl J Med 2005;353(20):2135–47.

70. Curtin JA, Busam K, Pinkel D, et al. Somatic activation of KIT in distinct subtypes of melanoma. J Clin Oncol 2006;24(26):4340–6.

71. Lens MB, Nathan P, Bataille V. Excision margins for primary cutaneous melanoma: updated pooled analysis of randomized controlled trials. Arch Surg 2007;142(9):885–91.

72. Easson AM, Rotstein LE, McCready DR. Lymph node assessment in melanoma. J Surg Oncol 2009;99:176–85.

73. Sasse AD, Sasse EC, Clark LGO, et al. Chemoimmunotherapy versus chemotherapy for metastatic malignant melanoma. Cochrane Database Syst Rev 2007;(1):CD005413. DOI:10.1002/14651858.CD005413.pub2.

74. Agarwal-Antal N, Bowen GM, Gerwels JW. Histologic evaluation of lentigo maligna with permanent sections: implications regarding current guidelines. J Am Acad Dermatol 2002;47:743–8.

75. Smalberger GJ, Siegel DM, Khachemoune A. Lentigo maligna. Dermatol Ther 2008;21(6):439–46.

76. Toker C. Trabecular carcinoma of the skin. Arch Dermatol 1972;105:107–10.

77. Tang CK, Toker C. Trabecular carcinoma of the skin: an ultrastructural study. Cancer 1978;42:2311–21.

78. Agelli C, Clegg LX. Epidemiology of primary Merkel cell carcinoma in the United States. J Am Acad Dermatol 2003;49:832–41.

79. Feng H, Shuda M, Chang Y, et al. Clonal integration of a polyomavirus in human Merkel cell carcinoma. Science 2008;319(5866):1096–100.

80. Andea AA, Coit DG, Amin B, et al. Merkel cell carcinoma: histologic features and prognosis. Cancer 2008;113(9):2549–58.

81. Henness S, Vereecken P. Management of Merkel tumours: an evidence-based review. Curr Opin Oncol 2008;20(3):280–6.

82. Yugueros P, Kane WJ, Goellner JR. Sweat gland carcinoma: a clinicopathologic analysis of an expanded series in a single institution. Plast Reconstr Surg 1998;102(3):705–10.

83. Ohta M, Hiramoto M, Ohtsuka H. Metastatic microcystic adnexal carcinoma: an autopsy case. Dermatol Surg 2004;30(6):957–60.

84. Gabillot-Carre M, Weill F, Mamelle G, et al. Microcystic adnexal carcinoma: report of seven cases including one with lung metastasis. Dermatology 2006;212(3): 221–8.

85. Breiting L, Christensen L, Dahlstrøm K, et al. Primary mucinous carcinoma of the skin: a population-based study. Int J Dermatol 2008;47(3):242–5.

86. Marra DE, Schanbacher CF, Torres A. Mohs micrographic surgery of primary cutaneous mucinous carcinoma using immunohistochemistry for margin control. Dermatol Surg 2004;30(5):799–802.

87. Frey J, Shimek C, Woodmansee C, et al. Aggressive digital papillary adenocarcinoma: a report of two diseases and review of the literature. J Am Acad Dermatol 2009;60(2):331–9.

88. Duke WH, Sherrod TT, Lupton GP. Papillary adenocarcinoma (aggressive digital papillary carcinoma revisited). Am J Surg Pathol 2000;24:775–84.

Skin Manifestations of Internal Disease

Andrew G. Franks, Jr., MD, FACP[a,b,c],*

KEYWORDS

- Autoimmune disease • Internal disease
- Connective tissue disease • Skin disorders

Internal disease can manifest in a myriad of skin dermatoses. This article provides descriptions, diagnostic methods, and possible treatments for some of these.

CALCIPHYLAXIS

Calciphylaxis is a syndrome characterized by small- and medium-sized vessel calcification and ischemic necrosis of skin and subcutaneous tissue due to stenotic fibrosis within the vessel wall.[1] It occurs predominantly in chronic renal failure with dialysis and may be associated with secondary hyperparathyroidism and an imbalance in calcium-phosphate metabolism.[2] Other causes include primary hyper-parathyroidism, diabetes, alcoholic liver disease, and connective tissue disease.[3] It may also occur in hypervitaminosis D, hypercalcemia of malignancy, warfarin use, and necrotizing vasculitis.[4] Clinical features include painful, violaceous, purpuric discoloration of the skin with subsequent retiform necrotic ulceration in a proximal or distal distribution (**Fig. 1**).[5] The pathogenesis is poorly understood, but reduction of protein C and protein S levels in some patients increases the probability of occurrence. Biopsy from an early lesion may reveal fine calcification of the vessel wall with subtle fibroblastic endovascular changes, but frank fibrosis and ischemia are usually absent.[6] Mature lesions reveal extensive calcification of the vessel wall along with proliferative endovascular fibrosis leading to tissue ischemia with necrosis of soft tissue and muscle.[7] The differential diagnosis includes thrombotic atheroemboli, cryoglobulinemia or cryofibrinogenemia, antiphospholipid syndrome, and vasculitis.

[a] Department of Dermatology, New York University School of Medicine, 550 First Avenue, New York, NY 10016, USA
[b] Division of Rheumatology, Department of Medicine, New York University School of Medicine, 550 First Avenue, New York, NY 10016, USA
[c] Skin Lupus & Connective Tissue Disease Section, New York University School of Medicine, 550 First Avenue, New York, NY 10016, USA
* Department of Dermatology, New York University School of Medicine, 550 First Avenue, New York, NY 10016.
E-mail address: andrew.franks@nyumc.org

Med Clin N Am 93 (2009) 1265–1282
doi:10.1016/j.mcna.2009.08.010
0025-7125/09/$ – see front matter © 2009 Published by Elsevier Inc.

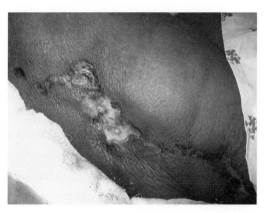

Fig. 1. Calciphylaxis.

Treatment has included normalization of serum calcium and phosphorus levels, correction of underlying clotting abnormalities, and avoiding subcutaneous trauma. Parathyroidectomy has been advocated if parathyroid hormone levels are elevated and hyperbaric oxygen therapy has been attempted but has generally been ineffective. Intravenous sodium thiosulfate and bisphosphonates have reportedly helped some patients.[8]

CHOLESTEROL EMBOLISM

The earliest signs of cholesterol embolism often are cutaneous, and are useful in identifying this under-diagnosed and potentially fatal condition.[9] Cholesterol embolization is a multisystem disorder because of the distal showering of cholesterol crystals usually occurring after aortic angiography, cardiac catheterization, coronary artery bypass graft surgery, percutaneous transluminal coronary angioplasty, other major vessel surgery, or anticoagulation.[10] Symptoms may be absent, unrecognized, or mimic other disease processes.[11] The primary sites of involvement are the kidney, followed by the skin and the gastrointestinal tract.[12] Cholesterol embolism is more common in male patients with significant atherosclerotic disease, hypertension, diabetes, and a history of tobacco use.[13] It is clinically characterized by livedo reticularis, leg pain, normal peripheral pulses, and acute renal failure.[14] The presentation may be atypical, with fever, myalgias, gastrointestinal bleeding, and multiorgan involvement mimicking systemic necrotizing vasculitis and thus often is not identified. The diagnosis should be strongly considered in elderly male patients with atherosclerotic vascular disease who have the onset of renal insufficiency with or without cutaneous manifestations after an invasive vascular procedure.[15] Livedo reticularis is a mottling of the skin in a bluish, lace-like pattern and is the most common cutaneous manifestation. It is usually bilateral and usually involves the feet and legs, extending to the thighs, trunk, and rarely the upper extremities (**Fig. 2**). Cyanosis, purpura, subcutaneous nodules, and ulcers can also be present. Gangrene may develop on the toes and eventually may require surgical debridement. Acrocyanosis or blue toe syndrome is a characteristic blue-black or violaceous discoloration of the toes and feet. The lesions are painful as the color change is secondary to decreased blood supply with tissue ischemia (**Fig. 3**). Indurated papules or nodules may appear on the thighs, legs, feet, and toes because of an inflammatory reaction surrounding cholesterol crystals. Purpura is most commonly seen on the legs and

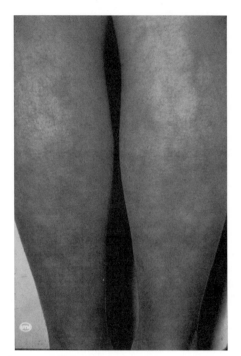

Fig. 2. Livedo reticularis.

the feet. The most common noncutaneous findings are fever, myalgias, gastrointestinal bleeding, altered mental status, and sudden onset arterial hypertension with renal failure. Most patients present with leg pain and livedo reticularis or blue toes in the presence of good peripheral pulses. Although peripheral hypereosinophilia may be

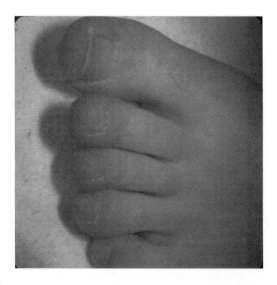

Fig. 3. Gangrene.

found, laboratory tests are not specific.[16] Skin, muscle, or renal biopsy demonstrating needle-shaped cholesterol clefts in intravascular microthrombi within small arteries and arterioles are the most specific finding. Medical therapy has generally been unsuccessful as treatment options are limited. Statin therapy for stabilizing plaques has been suggested anecdotally, but no definitive conclusion can be made.[17] Morbidity and mortality in patients with cholesterol emboli syndrome are high.[18] Death most often occurs from cardiovascular causes. Renal failure often progresses to dependence on dialysis.[19] Gangrene necessitating amputation is the major cutaneous complication of cholesterol embolization.[10] End diastolic pneumatic boot has been recommended in selected patients.[20] Surgery to remove the source of embolization using thromboaspiration, embolectomy, angioplasty, or blood vessel bypass may be the only remaining option.

CRYOGLOBULINEMIA

Cryoglobulins are abnormal immunoglobulins that form complexes and precipitate out of serum at low temperatures and redissolve upon warming or returning to room temperature. Studies have shown that the temperature at which cryoglobulins precipitate varies with the total cryoprotein concentration.[20] Higher concentrations of protein increase the temperature at which cryoglobulins precipitate. Positive test results with cryoglobulin concentrations greater than 1 mg/mL are indicative of active disease.[21] Cryoglobulins are made up of monoclonal antibodies immunoglobulin (Ig) M or IgG, rarely IgA.[22] IgM tends to precipitate at lower temperatures than does IgG cryoglobulin. Occasionally, IgM macroglobulin is both cryoprecipitable and capable of cold-induced antibody mediated agglutination of red cells. These are referred to as cold agglutinins. Not all cryoglobulins are cold agglutinins because they do not share some of the antibody characteristics of cold agglutinins. Several types of cryoglobulins have been identified, and the potential clinical manifestations vary by cryoglobulin type. When positive, the exact composition of protein is best detected by immunofixation electrophoresis.

Cryoglobulins are classified into three types based on their composition.[23] Type I cryoglobulinemia is made up of a monoclonal, homogeneous immunoglobulin usually IgM or less often IgG, IgA, or immunoglobulin light chains.[24] The cryoglobulin concentration is usually high, greater than 5 mg/mL. Examples of diseases associated with Type I cryoglobulinemia include Waldenström macroglobulinemia, paroxysmal cold hemoglobinuria, and other lymphoproliferative disorders. Types II and III cryoglobulinemia (mixed cryoglobulinemia) contain rheumatoid factors (RFs), which are usually IgM and, rarely, IgG or IgA. These RFs form complexes with the Fc portion of polyclonal IgG. The actual RF may be monoclonal (in type II cryoglobulinemia) or polyclonal (in type III cryoglobulinemia) immunoglobulin. Types II and III cryoglobulinemia represent 80% of all cryoglobulins. The cryoglobulin concentration is usually low—just above 1 mg/mL.

Types II and III, are called mixed cryoglobulinemias, and are associated with chronic inflammatory states such as systemic lupus erythematosus (SLE), Sjögren syndrome, and viral infections, particularly HCV.[25] Cutaneous vasculitis associated with cryoglobulinemia and hypocomplementemia is common in the course of chronic active hepatitis C infection. The triad of necrotizing vasculitis, chronic hepatitis C infection, and cryoglobulinemia occurs late after initial infection with hepatitis C. In these disorders, the IgG fraction is always polyclonal with either monoclonal (type II) or polyclonal (type III) IgM (rarely IgA or IgG) with RF activity.[26]

Cutaneous findings in cryoglobulinemia include erythematous to purpuric macules, papules and urticarial plaques, livedo reticularis, acral necrotic infarction, hemorrhagic erosions, painful distal ulcers and extensive post inflammatory hyperpigmentation (**Fig. 4**).[27] Lesions on the legs were common in all types of cryoglobulinemia; however, lesions on the head and mucosal surfaces of the nose and mouth more likely represent type I cryoglobulinemia. Skin biopsy most often reveals small vessel leukocytoclastic vasculitis and less frequently inflammatory or noninflammatory purpura, noninflammatory hyaline thrombosis, and postinflammatory sequelae.

CUTANEOUS SMALL VESSEL VASCULITIS

Inflammation and necrosis of blood vessels characterizes a broad spectrum of disorders that fall under the general category of vasculitis. Vasculitis may involve any size blood vessel, and vessel size is a useful way of classification.

Cutaneous small vessel vasculitis is most often associated with a heterogeneous group of disorders that include: drug hypersensitivity[28]; infections such as beta-hemolytic streptococcus, mycoplasma, Hepatitis B & C, and HIV; autoimmune disorders such as rheumatoid arthritis, SLE, Crohn disease; and malignancy, particularly of hematopoietic origin.[29,30] Skin biopsy reveals inflammation of the small blood vessels that is most prominent in the postcapillary venules.[31] This damage results in the most characteristic clinical finding of palpable purpura. However, early lesions may only be nonblanching petechiae or may be urticaria-like. Pustular, bullous, or ulcerated lesions may also develop and are commonly found on the ankles and lower legs. Residual postinflammatory hyperpigmentation usually occurs.[32]

Urticarial vasculitis (**Fig. 5**) is a distinctive syndrome usually characterized by persistent urticarial lesions, sometimes angioedema, arthralgias or arthritis, abdominal or chest pain, and may include pulmonary or renal involvement.[33] Clinical features that distinguish the skin lesions of urticarial vasculitis from allergic urticaria include: burning or pain rather than pruritus, individual lesions that resolve more slowly than allergic hives and usually take a few days to disappear as opposed to allergic urticaria where crops resolve within 24 hours, and significant postinflammatory hyperpigmentation.[34,35]

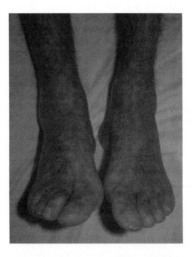

Fig. 4. Cryoglobulinemia.

Fig. 5. Urticarial vasculitis.

Henoch-Schönlein purpura (HSP) is a subset of small vessel vasculitis character-ized by intermittent purpura, arthralgias, abdominal pain, and renal disease. HSP is the most common vasculitis of childhood, but adult cases also occur and are prob-ably underrecognized. Purpura often appears on the extensor surfaces of the extremities (**Fig. 6**). They become hemorrhagic within a day or so and subsequently fade within a week with new crops appearing over a few weeks.[36] A viral infection or streptococcal pharyngitis is the usual triggering event. The cutaneous manifesta-tions are often preceded by mild fever, headache, and joint and abdominal pain. Pulmonary hemorrhage, abdominal pain, and gastrointestinal bleeding may occur at any time. Glomerulonephritis is the most common long-term component of the illness.[37]

LIVEDO RETICULARIS

Although primary livedo reticularis may be a benign, idiopathic condition, especially in young women, it may also be secondary to a wide variety of disorders whose common abnormality is thrombophilia—the increased tendency for the blood to clot.[38] These include anticardiolipin syndrome, connective tissue diseases such as SLE and rheumatoid arthritis, and malignancy.[39] Sneddon syndrome refers to livedo reticularis in association with CNS, eye, or heart involvement.[40] A violaceous lace-like network over the superficial plexus of vessels, is common on the legs, but may be more extensive in some patients.[41] The lesions usually do not blanch on diascopy. Livedo reticularis may disappear after several minutes in the prone position, thus having patients stand for a few minutes before the examination is an important diagnostic prerequisite. A number of different terms are used to

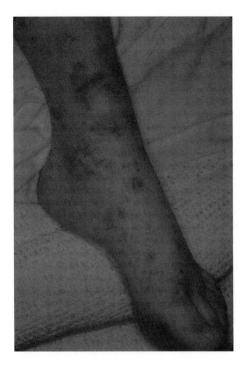

Fig. 6. Purpura.

describe the same or similar lesions including livedo or livedoid vasculopathy, and livedo or livedoid vasculitis.[42] The latter is often used when painful ulcerations occur about the ankles leading to atrophe blanche, a type of ulcer that heals with atrophic, white centers (**Fig. 7**).

THE NEUTROPHILIC DERMATOSES

The neutrophilic dermatoses are a spectrum of distinct clinical diseases characterized by sterile neutrophilic cutaneous infiltrates.[43] The cause of these disorders is not well understood but is thought to be related to deposition of immune complexes in dermal

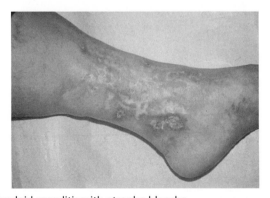

Fig. 7. Livedo or livedoid vasculitis with atrophe blanche.

vessels, resulting in complement fixation and leukocytoclastic vasculitis and altered neutrophilic chemotaxis.[44] The neutrophilic dermatoses include: erythema elevatum diutinum (EED), pyoderma gangrenosum (PG), Sneddon-Wilkinson disease, and Sweet syndrome.[45]

EED

EED is characterized by multiple symmetric papules, plaques, nodules, vesicles, or bullae on the extensor surface of joints, particularly the elbows, knees, hands, and feet. The lesions usually are initially red to purple in color, some becoming yellowish brown as they mature (**Fig. 8**). Many patients are asymptomatic but pruritus, tenderness, and pain may occur. They may be cold induced and demonstrate koebnerization. Constitutional symptoms may include arthralgias and fever. The course of the disease is chronic and frequently relapsing, though it may spontaneously remit. Lesions heal with residual atrophic patches with loss of collagen in the dermis.[46]

EED has been associated with a variety of underlying disorders such as rheumatoid arthritis and SLE,[47] in addition to HIV, hepatitis B, hepatitis C, mixed cryoglobulinemia, monoclonal gammopathy of undetermined significance (MGUS) particularly of the IgA type, myeloma, myelodysplasia, and leukemia.[48] Skin biopsy is not specific and usually reveals a dense perivascular neutrophilic infiltrate involving the superficial and mid dermis with leukocytoclastic vasculitis, fibrin deposition and endothelial swelling. An interstitial infiltrate of lymphocytes, neutrophils, eosinophils, plasma cells and histiocytes may be observed. Features of older lesions include perivascular fibrosis, intracellular lipid deposition, and capillary proliferation.[49] The treatment of choice for EED is dapsone. Other therapies reported in the literature include colchicine, topical, intralesional and systemic glucocorticoids, sulfapyridine, and chloroquine.

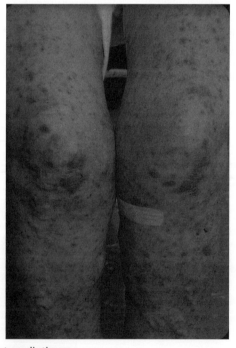

Fig. 8. Erythema elevatum diutinum.

PG

PG (**Fig. 9**) usually begins as painful papules or pustules that rapidly expand into painful burrowing ulcers with undermined borders and raised violaceous rims. The pretibial areas of the legs are the most frequent site, but any location may be involved. Different clinical presentations of PG include ulceration with a rapidly evolving purulent wound; discrete pustules, commonly associated with inflammatory bowel disease; superficial bullae with development of ulcerations; and vegetative erosions and superficial ulcers. An oral form of the disease, known as pyostomatitis vegetans occurs primarily in patients with inflammatory bowel disease.[50] Often the lesions heal leaving a cribriform scar. Ulcerations of PG may occur after trauma or any injury to the skin, and the term "pathergy" is used to describe the process. PG occurs most often in association with inflammatory bowel disease, but also with any of the connective tissue diseases, MGUS, myeloma, MDS, leukemia, and lymphoma.[51] Culture-negative pulmonary infiltrates are the most common extracutaneous manifestation. Histopathologic changes vary where the biopsy is taken in relation to the lesion but are not pathognomonic. Lymphocytic vasculitis is found in the area of erythema peripheral to the central ulceration, whereas neutrophilic infiltrates and abscess formation are identified more centrally. Dapsone, thalidomide, intravenous gamma globulin, systemic steroids, and tumor necrosis factor-α inhibitors have been used in therapy.[52,53]

Sneddon-Wilkinson Disease

Sneddon-Wilkinson disease, or subcorneal pustular dermatosis, is a recurrent, pustular disorder that may mimic pustular psoriasis or inverse psoriasis, and presents with bilateral crops of lesions on the flanks, trunk, and proximal extremities with a flexural tendency (**Fig. 10**).[54] The primary lesions are pea-sized sterile pustules

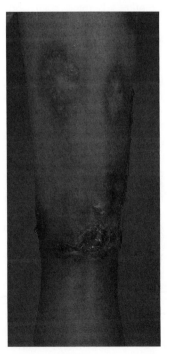

Fig. 9. Pyoderma gangrenosum.

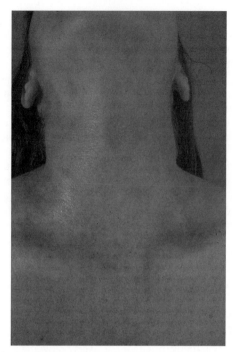

Fig. 10. Sneddon-Wilkinson disease.

and papulovesicles often described as half-pustular (bottom) and half-clear (top) or "half and half blister."[55] Sometimes burning, pain, and tenderness of the affected areas of the skin may occur. Subsequently, the lesions may coalesce and form annular polycyclic rings, which eventually crust and erode. The histopathology reveals a subcorneal pustule filled with polymorphonuclear leukocytes with only occasional eosinophils and absence of spongiosis and acantholysis. Constitutional features may not be prominent, but generalized arthralgias and arthritis may occur. It is frequently associated with an MGUS, particularly IgA, less commonly IgG.[56] Multiple myeloma and other lymphoproliferative disorders are sometimes found and an association with PG has been noted.

Sweet Syndrome

The combination of high fever; leukocytosis; boggy, red, painful papules; and plaques with dense neutrophilic dermal infiltrates without evidence of vasculitis on skin biopsy is characteristic of Sweet syndrome, or acute febrile neutrophilic dermatosis.[57] Soft, pea-sized papules and papulovesicles grouped within a boggy violaceous plaque are very suggestive of the diagnosis. If the plaque is squeezed between the thumb and forefinger, a gray-yellow coloration may be noted within the papules (**Fig. 11**). Lesions tend to occur on the extremities more so than the trunk. Sweet syndrome may be associated with hematological malignancy,[58] especially acute myelogenous leukemia and inflammatory bowel disease, particularly Crohn disease.[59] The initial episode is often thought to be cellulitis or erysipelas, and patients are then placed on antibiotics empirically. As spontaneous remission usually occurs, the misdiagnosis is reinforced. Patients may become secondarily infected causing further confusion. SSKI is useful in patients when steroids fail or are contraindicated.

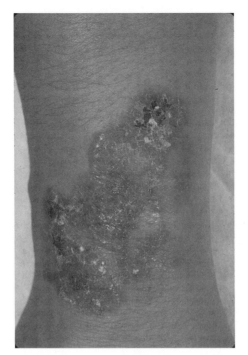

Fig. 11. Sweet syndrome.

RAYNAUD PHENOMENON

Many rheumatologic diseases are associated with Raynaud phenomenon, most commonly systemic sclerosis, of which it is often the initial manifestation. It may also occur in SLE, dermatomyositis, rheumatoid arthritis, and other autoimmune collagen vascular disorders.[60] Several noninflammatory conditions including hand-arm vibration syndrome,[61] thoracic outlet syndrome, paraproteinemia, and treatment with medications, especially beta-blockers and antineoplastic agents may also precipitate the disease. As distinguished from patients with secondary Raynaud phenomenon, patients with the primary form typically have a younger age of onset, normal nail fold capillaries, and negative or low titers of autoantibodies. Primary Raynaud phenomenon attacks typically involve all fingers in a symmetric fashion (**Fig. 12**), and are associated with minimal pain. By contrast, asymmetrical finger involvement and intense pain suggest underlying pathology. Both primary and secondary Raynaud phenomenon often, but not always, spare the thumbs.[62] Physical examination findings characteristic of secondary Raynaud phenomenon include digital tuft pits, necrotic changes, onycholysis, and pterygium inversum. Radial and brachial pulses are usually normal. Nail fold capillaries can be examined through an ophthalmoscope set at 20 to 40 diopters or with a handheld dermatoscope—both using clear surgical gel. The presence of tortuous and dilated capillaries and areas of "vessel dropout" indicative of avascularity, are characteristic of secondary Raynaud phenomenon.[63]

PALISADED NEUTROPHILIC AND GRANULOMATOUS DERMATITIS

Palisaded neutrophilic and granulomatous dermatitis is characterized by lesions that are usually symmetrically distributed on the extremities and have smooth, ulcerated,

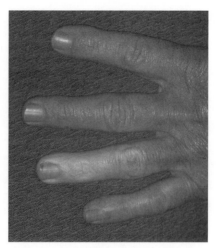

Fig. 12. Raynaud phenomenon.

or umbilicated surfaces (**Fig. 13**).[64] When fully formed, they often resemble "breakfast pastry" with elevated, crusty papular borders and central circular swirls. Previously, the term rheumatoid papule was used for single, small lesions, or Churg-Strauss granuloma, when larger and mature.[65] Palisaded granulomatous inflammation in the presence or absence of leukocytoclastic vasculitis is found on skin biopsy. It is usually associated with systemic immune-complex mediated disease, especially autoimmune conditions such as rheumatoid arthritis and SLE. It may spontaneously remit, but most patients respond to treatment of the underlying disease.[66]

MORPHEA

Morphea is not a single disease, but rather a reactive phenomenon with many different causes. There are probably autoimmune, infectious, and environmental types. Depending on the clinical situation, an underlying cause may sometimes be identified.

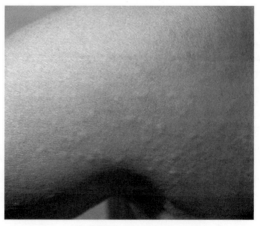

Fig. 13. Palisaded neutrophilic and granulomatous dermatitis.

Thus, a single plaque on the back of a young woman may remit spontaneously without incident with no identifiable cause, but multiple plaques, linear involvement, or progressive involvement may warrant further evaluation. Localized, generalized, guttate, Lichen sclerosis atrophicus-morphea overlap, linear, coup de sabre, and profundus are recognized categories and may overlap in some patients (**Fig. 14**). Various infections such as beta hemolytic streptococcus, Epstein-Barr virus, and Borrelia have been suggested. Radiation therapy and heavy metal poisoning have also been noted. The incipient phase of systemic sclerosis or overlap syndromes may begin with morphea. Only with time does the systemic nature of the disease uncover itself. Thus, caution is advised until appropriate studies to rule out systemic disease have been conducted. Treatments with doxycycline, hydroxychloroquine, colchicine, methotrexate, narrow band UV-B, and UV-A1 have been used.

TUMID LUPUS ERYTHEMATOSUS

Smooth, indurated, nonscarring, pink to violaceous papules, plaques, or nodules, devoid of surface changes which are usually distributed on sun-exposed sites are the clinical hallmarks of tumid lupus erythematosus (**Fig. 15**). Until recently, it was often not possible to differentiate tumid lupus erythematosus from other disorders with similar clinical and histopathologic presentations, such as polymorphous light eruption, lymphocytic infiltrate of Jessner and Kanof, pseudolymphoma, and deep gyrate erythema. Skin biopsy reveals a superficial and deep perivascular and periadnexal infiltrate of lymphocytes with few plasma cells. A colloidal iron or alcian blue stain shows increased extracellular mucin deposits within the papillary and reticular dermis. Junctional epidermal changes are minimal to absent. The CD4/CD8 ratio is usually equal to or greater than 3:1. Direct immunofluorescence is usually negative, coinciding with the absence of junctional change. Tumid lupus follows a chronic, benign, nonscarring course, and is classified as a form of chronic cutaneous lupus erythematosus. Just as in other forms of chronic cutaneous lupus, it may be a cutaneous feature of SLE. Atypical cutaneous mucinosis with T-cell lymphoma may require gene rearrangement studies to clarify.

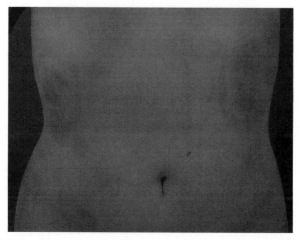

Fig. 14. Morphea.

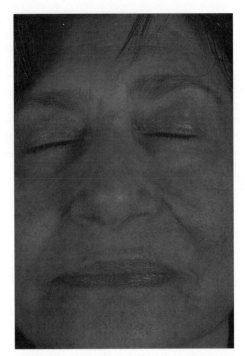

Fig. 15. Tumid lupus erythematosus.

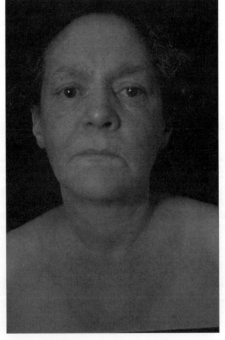

Fig. 16. Amyopathic dermatomyositis.

AMYOPATHIC DERMATOMYOSITIS

Amyopathic dermatomyositis by definition demonstrates the typical cutaneous findings of dermatomyositis without muscular weakness or elevation of muscle enzymes for a minimum of 2 years. Patients who have already received therapy with high-dose corticosteroids or immunosuppressive agents are not included in this category. Subclinical muscle involvement may occur in some patients and may be demonstrated by ultrasound, CT, MRI, electromyography, or muscle biopsy. The clinical cutaneous hallmarks include malar rash, which usually targets the nasolabial fold (in SLE it is usually spared) and is associated with perioral sparing (**Fig. 16**); heliotrope eruption of the eyelids; shawl sign over the posterior neck and shoulders; holster sign over the trochanteric areas of the thighs; linear extensor erythema, which when on the hand may obscure Gottron papules and sign; Gottron papules and sign over the interphalangeal and metacarpal joints, and elbows and knees; and, periungual suffusion with areas of tortuous vessels, "vascular dropout," and cuticular disarray. The incidence of pulmonary fibrosis and underlying malignancy is similar to those patients with overt muscle disease.

ACKNOWLEDGMENT

Dr Franks would like to thank Theresa Repetti for her extensive and skilled assistance in preparing this article for publication.

REFERENCES

1. Bazari H, Jaff MR, Mannstadt M, et al. Case records of the Massachusetts General Hospital. Case 7–2007. A 59-year-old woman with diabetic renal disease and nonhealing skin ulcers. N Engl J Med 2007;356(10):1049–57.
2. Dauden E, Onate MJ. Calciphylaxis. Dermatol Clin 2008;26(4):557–68, ix.
3. Nigwekar SU, Wolf M, Sterns RH, et al. Calciphylaxis from nonuremic causes: a systematic review. Clin J Am Soc Nephrol 2008;3(4):1139–43.
4. Lee JL, Naguwa SM, Cheema G, et al. Recognizing calcific uremic arteriolopathy in autoimmune disease: an emerging mimicker of vasculitis. Autoimmun Rev 2008;7(8):638–43.
5. Bosler DS, Amin MB, Gulli F, et al. Unusual case of calciphylaxis associated with metastatic breast carcinoma. Am J Dermatopathol 2007;29(4):400–3.
6. Weenig RH, Sewell LD, Davis MD, et al. Calciphylaxis: natural history, risk factor analysis, and outcome. J Am Acad Dermatol 2007;56(4):569–79.
7. Reed KB, Davis MD. The incidence of physician-diagnosed calciphylaxis: a population-based study. J Am Acad Dermatol 2007;57(2):365–6.
8. Rogers NM, Coates PT. Calcific uraemic arteriolopathy: an update. Curr Opin Nephrol Hypertens 2008;17(6):629–34.
9. Jucgla A, Moreso F, Muniesa C, et al. Cholesterol embolism: still an unrecognized entity with a high mortality rate. J Am Acad Dermatol 2006;55(5):786–93.
10. Meyrier A. Cholesterol crystal embolism: diagnosis and treatment. Kidney Int 2006;69(8):1308–12.
11. Mittal BV, Alexander MP, Rennke HG, et al. Atheroembolic renal disease: a silent masquerader. Kidney Int 2008;73(1):126–30.
12. McCullough PA, Adam A, Becker CR, et al. Epidemiology and prognostic implications of contrast-induced nephropathy. Am J Cardiol 2006;98(6A):5K–13K.
13. Olin JW. Atheroembolic renal disease: underdiagnosed and misunderstood. Catheter Cardiovasc Interv 2007;70(6):789–90.

14. Brewster UC. Dermatological disease in patients with CKD. Am J Kidney Dis 2008;51(2):331–44.
15. Hitti WA, Wali RK, Weinman EJ, et al. Cholesterol embolization syndrome induced by thrombolytic therapy. Am J Cardiovasc Drugs 2008;8(1):27–34.
16. Cecioni I, Fassio F, Gori S, et al. Eosinophilia in cholesterol atheroembolic disease. J Allergy Clin Immunol 2007;120(6):1470–1 [author reply 1471].
17. Molisse TA, Tunick PA, Kronzon I. Complications of aortic atherosclerosis: atheroemboli and thromboemboli. Curr Treat Options Cardiovasc Med 2007;9(2): 137–47.
18. Scolari F, Ravani P, Gaggi R, et al. The challenge of diagnosing atheroembolic renal disease: clinical features and prognostic factors. Circulation 2007;116(3): 298–304.
19. Sarwar S, Al-Absi A, Wall BM. Catastrophic cholesterol crystal embolization after endovascular stent placement for peripheral vascular disease. Am J Med Sci 2008;335(5):403–6.
20. Vermeersch P, Gijbels K, Knockaert D, et al. Establishment of reference values for immunoglobulins in the cryoprecipitate. Clin Immunol 2008;129(2):360–4.
21. Shihabi ZK. Cryoglobulins: an important but neglected clinical test. Ann Clin Lab Sci 2006;36(4):395–408.
22. Ferri C. Mixed cryoglobulinemia. Orphanet J Rare Dis 2008;3:25.
23. Tedeschi A, Baratè C, Minola E, et al. Cryoglobulinemia. Blood Rev 2007;21(4): 183–200.
24. Yagi Y, Tanioka M, Kambe N, et al. Cryogloblinaemia type I: serum cryoprecipitate formation at 25 degrees C. Clin Exp Dermatol 2008;33(3):361–2.
25. Sansonno D, Carbone A, De Re V, et al. Hepatitis C virus infection, cryoglobulinaemia, and beyond. Rheumatology (Oxford) 2007;46(4):572–8.
26. Ramos-Casals M, Robles A, Brito-Zerón P, et al. Life-threatening cryoglobulinemia: clinical and immunological characterization of 29 cases. Semin Arthritis Rheum 2006;36(3):189–96.
27. Requena L, Kutzner H, Angulo J, et al. Generalized livedo reticularis associated with monoclonal cryoglobulinemia and multiple myeloma. J Cutan Pathol 2007; 34(2):198–202.
28. Bahrami S, Malone JC, Webb KG, et al. Tissue eosinophilia as an indicator of drug-induced cutaneous small-vessel vasculitis. Arch Dermatol 2006;142(2): 155–61.
29. Carlson JA, Chen KR. Cutaneous vasculitis update: small vessel neutrophilic vasculitis syndromes. Am J Dermatopathol 2006;28(6):486–506.
30. Lotti T, Ghersetich I, Comacchi C, et al. Cutaneous small-vessel vasculitis. J Am Acad Dermatol 1998;39(5 Pt 1):667–87 [quiz 688–90].
31. Guha B, Youngberg G, Krishnaswamy G. Urticaria and urticarial vasculitis. Compr Ther 2003;29(2–3):146–56.
32. Russell JP, Gibson LE. Primary cutaneous small vessel vasculitis: approach to diagnosis and treatment. Int J Dermatol 2006;45(1):3–13.
33. Brown NA, Carter JD. Urticarial vasculitis. Curr Rheumatol Rep 2007;9(4):312–9.
34. Chang S, Carr W. Urticarial vasculitis. Allergy Asthma Proc 2007;28(1):97–100.
35. Venzor J, Lee WL, Huston DP. Urticarial vasculitis. Clin Rev Allergy Immunol 2002; 23(2):201–16.
36. Roberts PF, Waller TA, Brinker TM, et al. Henoch-Schonlein purpura: a review article. Southampt Med J 2007;100(8):821–4.
37. Fretzayas A, Sionti I, Moustaki M, et al. Henoch-Schonlein purpura: a long-term prospective study in Greek children. J Clin Rheumatol 2008;14(6):324–31.

38. Gibbs MB, 3rd English JC, Zirwas MJ. Livedo reticularis: an update. J Am Acad Dermatol 2005;52(6):1009–19.
39. Toubi E, Shoenfeld Y. Livedo reticularis as a criterion for antiphospholipid syndrome. Clin Rev Allergy Immunol 2007;32(2):138–44.
40. Legierse CM, Canninga-Van Dijk MR, Bruijnzeel-Koomen CA, et al. Sneddon syndrome and the diagnostic value of skin biopsies—three young patients with intracerebral lesions and livedo racemosa. Eur J Dermatol 2008;18(3): 322–8.
41. Fleischer AB Jr, Resnick SD. Livedo reticularis. Dermatol Clin 1990;8(2):347–54.
42. Calamia KT, Balabanova M, Perniciaro C, et al. Livedo (livedoid) vasculitis and the factor V Leiden mutation: additional evidence for abnormal coagulation. J Am Acad Dermatol 2002;46(1):133–7.
43. Saavedra AP, Kovacs SC, Moschella SL. Neutrophilic dermatoses. Clin Dermatol 2006;24(6):470–81.
44. Wallach D. [Neutrophilic dermatoses]. Rev Med Interne 2005;26(1):41–53.
45. Callen JP. Neutrophilic dermatoses. Dermatol Clin 2002;20(3):409–19.
46. Wahl CE, Bouldin MB, Gibson LE. Erythema elevatum diutinum: clinical, histopathologic, and immunohistochemical characteristics of six patients. Am J Dermatopathol 2005;27(5):397–400.
47. Bouaziz JD, Barete S, Le Pelletier F, et al. Cutaneous lesions of the digits in systemic lupus erythematosus: 50 cases. Lupus 2007;16(3):163–7.
48. Ayoub N, Charuel JL, Diemert MC, et al. Antineutrophil cytoplasmic antibodies of IgA class in neutrophilic dermatoses with emphasis on erythema elevatum diutinum. Arch Dermatol 2004;140(8):931–6.
49. Crowson AN, Jr Mihm MC, Magro CM. Cutaneous vasculitis: a review. J Cutan Pathol 2003;30(3):161–73.
50. Davis MD, Nakamura KJ. Peristomal pyoderma gangrenosum associated with collagenous colitis. Arch Dermatol 2007;143(5):669–70.
51. Callen JP, Jackson JM. Pyoderma gangrenosum: an update. Rheum Dis Clin North Am 2007;33(4):787–802, vi.
52. Kreuter A, Reich-Schupke S, Stücker M, et al. Intravenous immunoglobulin for pyoderma gangrenosum. Br J Dermatol 2008;158(4):856–7.
53. Adisen E, Oztas M, Gurer MA. Treatment of idiopathic pyoderma gangrenosum with infliximab: induction dosing regimen or on-demand therapy? Dermatology 2008;216(2):163–5.
54. Bordignon M, Zattra E, Montesco MC, et al. Subcorneal pustular dermatosis (Sneddon-Wilkinson disease) with absence of desmoglein 1 and 3 antibodies: case report and literature review. Am J Clin Dermatol 2008;9(1):51–5.
55. Cheng S, Edmonds E, Ben-Gashir M, et al. Subcorneal pustular dermatosis: 50 years on. Clin Exp Dermatol 2008;33(3):229–33.
56. Launay F, Albès B, Bayle P, et al. [Sneddon-Wilkinson disease. Four cases report]. Rev Med Interne 2004;25(2):154–9.
57. Cohen PR. Sweet's syndrome—a comprehensive review of an acute febrile neutrophilic dermatosis. Orphanet J Rare Dis 2007;2:34.
58. Buck T, González LM, Lambert WC, et al. Sweet's syndrome with hematologic disorders: a review and reappraisal. Int J Dermatol 2008;47(8):775–82.
59. Ratzinger G, Burgdorf W, Zelger BG, et al. Acute febrile neutrophilic dermatosis: a histopathologic study of 31 cases with review of literature. Am J Dermatopathol 2007;29(2):125–33.
60. Bakst R, Merola JF, Franks AG Jr, et al. Raynaud's phenomenon: pathogenesis and management. J Am Acad Dermatol 2008;59(4):633–53.

61. Youakim S. The validity of Raynaud's phenomenon symptoms in HAVS cases. Occup Med (Lond) 2008;58(6):431–5.
62. Chikura B, Moore TL, Manning JB, et al. Sparing of the thumb in Raynaud's phenomenon. Rheumatology (Oxford) 2008;47(2):219–21.
63. Ingegnoli F, Boracchi P, Gualtierotti R, et al. Prognostic model based on nailfold capillaroscopy for identifying Raynaud's phenomenon patients at high risk for the development of a scleroderma spectrum disorder: PRINCE (prognostic index for nailfold capillaroscopic examination). Arthritis Rheum 2008;58(7):2174–82.
64. Bremner R, Simpson E, White CR, et al. Palisaded neutrophilic and granulomatous dermatitis: an unusual cutaneous manifestation of immune-mediated disorders. Semin Arthritis Rheum 2004;34(3):610–6.
65. Sangueza OP, Caudell MD, Mengesha YM, et al. Palisaded neutrophilic granulomatous dermatitis in rheumatoid arthritis. J Am Acad Dermatol 2002;47(2):251–7.
66. Hantash BM, Chiang D, Kohler S, et al. Palisaded neutrophilic and granulomatous dermatitis associated with limited systemic sclerosis. J Am Acad Dermatol 2008;58(4):661–4.

Update on Cutaneous Manifestations of Infectious Diseases

Dirk M. Elston, MD

KEYWORDS

- MRSA • Staphylococcus • Monkey pox • Mycobacteria
- Fungal • Chikungunya

BACTERIAL INFECTIONS

Community-acquired, methicillin-resistant *Staphylococcus aureus* (CA-MRSA) has emerged as the most important new bacterial pathogen for dermatologists because of its tendency to present with furunculosis and abscesses.[1] Large outbreaks often occur in daycare centers and among members of athletic teams, and CA-MRSA has moved into hospitals and become a major cause of hospital-acquired sepsis.[2] CA-MRSA infections can be particularly severe in children, where life-threatening pneumonitis, lytic bone lesions, and other systemic complications can occur.[3,4] Multi-drug-resistant strains are emerging and the widespread use of drugs, such as tetracycline, in animal feed may contribute to the emergence of resistance.[5]

The majority of CA-MRSA abscesses will respond to drainage.[6–9] A systemic antibiotic should be used when there is evidence of sepsis or invasion into adjacent tissues, and decolonization is reasonable when there is evidence of spread to other members of a family or other close contacts. Any attempt at decolonization must address both the skin and the nares because intervention aimed only at the nares often fail.[10] Bleach baths (two tablespoons of bleach per quarter tub), chlorhexidine, and triclosan remain effective for decolonization of moist intertriginous and eczematous skin. Mupirocin, retapamulin, triple antibiotic, and tea tree oil cream have all be used for nasal carriage, as have oral regimens of rifampin plus minocycline. Emerging clindamycin resistance makes nasal decolonization with this agent problematic in many areas.[11,12]

Most patients who require antibiotic therapy can be managed cost effectively with trimethoprim-sulfamethoxasole or a tetracycline. As noted earlier, emerging clindamycin resistance makes this antibiotic a more problematic choice. Inducible clindamycin resistance is particularly common among children with cystic fibrosis.[13]

Refractory and complicated skin infections often need newer antibiotics, including parenteral agents. According to the US Food and Drug Administration and the Centers

Department of Dermatology, Geisinger Medical Center, 100 North Academy Avenue, Danville, PA 17821, USA
E-mail address: Delston@geisinger.edu

Med Clin N Am 93 (2009) 1283–1290
doi:10.1016/j.mcna.2009.08.009
0025-7125/09/$ – see front matter © 2009 Published by Elsevier Inc.

medical.theclinics.com

for Disease Control, complicated skin infections are those that involve deeper soft tissue, require surgical intervention beyond simple incision and drainage, occur concurrently with systemic involvement; occur in the presence of a significant underlying disease state that complicates the response to treatment; occur in an anatomic site where the risk for anaerobic or gram-negative pathogen involvement is higher (eg, rectal area); occur from injury sustained in a wet environment where unusual pathogens are more likely; or occur as a result of a bite injury. Physical signs and symptoms suggesting more serious infection include rapid progression, pain out of proportion to physical findings, anesthesia, bullae, hemorrhage, slough or gas in tissue.

The treatment of complicated skin infections will generally require surgery in addition to an antibiotic. In this setting, antibiotic selection should generally be based on the results of culture and sensitivity, although in injuries resulting from bites, empiric therapy directed against *Pasteurella* species is appropriate. Drugs, such as oral amoxicillin/clavulanate, intravenous ampicillin/sulbactam, or ertapenem, are often used in this setting. Other organisms may occur in bite injuries, including *Staphylococcus aureus, Bacteroides* species, and *Capnocytophaga canimorsus.*

Therapeutic failure is being reported more commonly with vancomycin, and may relate intracellular survival of bacteria. This resistance can often be overcome by the addition of rifampin.[14] Fluoroquinolones provide inconsistent coverage against staphylococci, including CA-MRSA.[15,16] They remain appropriate for pseudomonas infections. Linezolid can be effective, even in wounds with compromised blood flow.[17]

Linezolid is an oxazolidinone. One of its outstanding characteristics is that is has almost 100% oral bioavailability. It has proved to be more reliable than vancomycin in the treatment of serious staphylococcal infections.[18–22] Daptomycin is a cyclic lipopeptide. It acts through disruption of bacterial membrane electrical potentials. Daptomycin has been used effectively in serious skin infections including CA-MRSA infections. It may be effective in some MRSA isolates with heteroresistance to vancomycin.[23–26] The drug can be dosed once daily. It is cleared renally, and is generally well tolerated, although there are some reports of myopathy and potential for adverse interactions with HMG-CoA reductase inhibitors. Resistance has been reported, and in vitro sensitivity testing may not always predict clinical outcome.[27–29] Tigecycline is an intravenous glycylcycline 9-tert-butyl-glycylamido derivative of minocycline. It has proved particularly useful for the treatment of infections involving MRSA and enteric organisms.[30] Unfortunately, it has minimal activity against *Pseudomonas aeruginosa* and *Proteus spp.*, but it may be effective in the treatment of serious infections caused by *Acinetobacter baumannii,* when few choices are available.[31]

Quinupristin-dalfopristin, a parental streptogramin, has been used effectively in some critically ill patients who have MRSA infections that failed to respond to vancomycin. Unfortunately, 31% of MRSA isolates are resistant in some areas.[32] Telavancin, a multivalent lipoglycopeptide derivative of vancomycin, demonstrates rapid bactericidal activity against CA-MRSA.[33] It has a long serum half-life, allowing once daily administration. Dalbavancin, a semisynthetic glycopeptide derivative of teicoplanin, has an even longer half-life allowing for weekly administration. In a randomized, controlled, double-blind trial, once-weekly dalbavancin was as effective as twice-daily linezolid. MRSA accounted for 51% of the cultured pathogens.[34] Carbapenems, such as panipenem, meropenem, and ertapenem, demonstrate broad-spectrum activity and synergism with vancomycin.[35,36] Their spectrum is too broad for most skin infections. Ceftobiprole medocaril is a parenteral cephalosporin active against MRSA.[37] In some studies, it compared favorably to vancomycin.[38] Small-colony variants of staphylococci may not be as susceptible to the drug.[39]

Vibrio vulnificus is often found in brackish water and causes serious infection in patients who have cirrhosis who sustain injuries in aquatic environments or consume raw oysters.[40] Marine *Vibrio* infection should be suspected in anyone with liver disease and cellulitis, hypotension, or sepsis.

Acinetobacter baumannii is an important emerging pathogen, causing severe systemic and soft-tissue infections, mostly in hospitalized patients. Some strains are resistant to almost all available antibiotics, but tend to be susceptible to carbapenems.[41]

MYCOBACTERIAL INFECTIONS

Tuberculosis and nontuberculous mycobacterial infections have emerged as important pathogens in patients who have iatrogenic immunosuppression, including therapy with biologic agents, in particular anti-TNF therapy.[42,43] Disseminated *Mycobacterium avium* complex infection, often associated with HIV infection, has also be reported in patients treated with infliximab.[44]

Severe skin infections with nontuberculous mycobacteria have been reported in association with nail salon foot baths or following mesotherapy.[45,46] Patients typically present with abscesses, deep draining sinus tracts, or furuncles.[47–49] *Mycobacterium chelonae* infections have been reported after liposuction.[50] Disseminated nontuberculous mycobacterial infection in Thai patients without HIV often demonstrate coinfection with other opportunistic pathogens, suggesting the possibility of a new transmissible AIDS like agent.[51]

Tuberculosis has also reemerged as an important disease, partly in relation to the HIV epidemic, and partly because of the widespread use of anti-TNF agents. Skin tests may fail to detect infection and patients who have signs or symptoms of infection may need imaging studies, interferon gamma release assays, or DNA hybridization studies.[52,53]

Clarithromycin has emerged as the best empiric choice for cutaneous nontuberculous mycobacterial infections.[54] Other agents that are often effective for *M. marinum* include minocycline or a combination of rifampin and ethambutol.[55–57]

M. abscessus infections generally need surgical and multidrug antimicrobial therapy with clarithromycin or azithromycin combined with amikacin.[58]

FUNGAL INFECTIONS

Zygomycosis (mucormycosis) is an increasing important pathogen because of its high morbidity and the rising prevalence of diabetes, the major risk factor for infection. The diagnosis is typically based on a biopsy specimen. The organism is vasculotropic and vasculodestructive and is visible in histologic sections as wide, brightly eosinophilic ribbons with hollow centers. Posaconazole is active against Zygomycetes and has improved the outlook for these infections.

Fusarium is replacing *Candida* and *Aspergillus* as fungal pathogens in immunocompromised hosts because of better prophylaxis that has decreased the incidence of the other two pathogens. Fusarium isolated from patients who are non-neutropenic and nonimmunosuppressed is rarely a pathogen, but in the setting of chemotherapy-induced neutropenia, the infection is often fatal.[59] As in *Candida* sepsis, fever and myalgia are typical presenting findings. Skin lesions typically present as leathery, black eschars with scalloped erythematous and edematous borders. The organism may be recovered from a skin biopsy or from blood cultures.[60] Fusariosis may also present with arthritis, onychomycosis, keratitis, or endophthalmitis.[61] The prognosis is poor despite amphotericin B therapy unless the neutropenia resolves. Newer agents, such as voriconazole, show activity against fusariosis.

Penicillium marneffei is an opportunistic dimorphic fungal pathogen endemic to Southeast Asia. It is being seen in patients who have AIDS who have traveled to endemic regions. Histopathologically, the organism closely resembles histoplasmosis.[62] Amphotericin B and itraconazole are active against *P. marneffei.*

Exserohilum, a dematiaceous fungus, has emerged as a cause of cutaneous, corneal, and sinus infection, especially in the southern United States. Aggressive debridement is critical, as the organism responds poorly to amphotericin B. The addition of a triazole antifungal may be of benefit.[63]

VIRAL INFECTIONS

Monkeypox emerged as an important pathogen in the Midwestern United States in 2003. The index case was a 3-year-old girl who developed fever and cellulitis after having been bitten by a prairie dog. The outbreak was traced to a single shipment of exotic animals from Ghana.[64] Clinical manifestations are similar to those of smallpox. After an incubation period of 5 to 21 days, the patient experiences headaches, fever, chills, sweats, and lymphadenopathy. This prodrome is followed in a couple of days by a vesiculopustular eruption. Individual lesions evolve from umbilicated pustules to hemorrhagic crusts. In contrast to smallpox, lesions are in various stages of evolution.

Just as monkey pox was important because of its clinical similarities to smallpox, Chikungunya virus is important because of its clinical similarities to Dengue.[65] Several outbreaks occurred recently in popular Indian Ocean resort islands. Travelers brought the infection home with them, and it has become established in countries like Italy where vectors already existed. Transmission is by way of Aedes aegypti mosquitoes that had spread to Italy from the United States. It is only a matter of time before the virus becomes endemic in parts of the United States. Infection typically presents with fever, arthralgia, myalgia, and rash. Atypical features, such as bullous lesions and genital ulceration, have been reported.[66,67] Other systemic features may include cardiovascular, neurologic, or respiratory involvement. The overall mortality is approximately10% and increases with age.

We have become a global village and diseases now spread easily from remote corners of the world. New medications, such as the biologics, offer dramatic results for our patients, but may be complicated by unusual infections. The dermatologist is on the front lines with these infections, as they typically present with cutaneous lesions.

REFERENCES

1. Wilson ME. The traveler and emerging infections: sentinel, courier, transmitter. J Appl Microbiol 2003;94(Suppl):1S–11S.
2. Shorr AF. Epidemiology and economic impact of methicillin-resistant *Staphylococcus aureus*: review and analysis of the literature. Pharmacoeconomics 2007;25(9):751–68.
3. Hoshino C, Satoh N, Sugawara S, et al. Community-acquired *Staphylococcus aureus* pneumonia accompanied by rapidly progressive glomerulonephritis and hemophagocytic syndrome. Intern Med 2007;46(13):1047–53.
4. Nourse C, Starr M, Munckhof W. Community-acquired methicillin-resistant *Staphylococcus aureus* causes severe disseminated infection and deep venous thrombosis in children: literature review and recommendations for management. J Paediatr Child Health 2007;43:656–61.

5. van Duijkeren E, Ikawaty R, Broekhuizen-Stins MJ, et al. Transmission of methi-cillin-resistant *Staphylococcus aureus* strains between different kinds of pig farms. Vet Microbiol 2008;126:383–9.

6. Rajendran PM, Young D, Maurer T, et al. Randomized, double-blind, placebo-controlled trial of cephalexin for treatment of uncomplicated skin abscesses in a population at risk for community methicillin-resistant *Staphylococcus aureus* infection. Antimicrob Agents Chemother 2007;51:4044–8.

7. Fridkin SK, Hageman JC, Morrison M, et al. Active bacterial core surveillance program of the emerging infections program network. methicillin-resistant *Staphylococcus aureus* disease in three communities. N Engl J Med 2005;352(14): 1436–44.

8. Lee MC, Rios AM, Aten MF, et al. Management and outcome of children with skin and soft tissue abscesses caused by community-acquired methicillin-resistant *Staphylococcus aureus*. Pediatr Infect Dis J 2004;23(2):123–7.

9. Young DM, Harris HW, Charlebois ED, et al. An epidemic of methicillin-resistant *Staphylococcus aureus* soft tissue infections among medically underserved patients. Arch Surg 2004;139(9):947–51.

10. Ellis MW, Griffith ME, Dooley DP, et al. Targeted intranasal mupirocin to prevent community-associated methicillin-resistant *Staphylococcus aureus* colonization and infection in soldiers: a cluster randomized controlled trial. Antimicrob Agents Chemother 2007;51:3591–8.

11. Seal JB, Moreira B, Bethel CD, et al. Antimicrobial resistance in *Staphylococcus aureus* at the University of Chicago Hospitals: a 15-year longitudinal assessment in a large university-based hospital. Infect Control Hosp Epidemiol 2003;24(6): 403–8.

12. Tsuji BT, Rybak MJ, Cheung CM, et al. Community- and health care-associated methicillin-resistant Staphylococcus aureus: a comparison of molecular epidemi-ology and antimicrobial activities of various agents. Diagn Microbiol Infect Dis 2007;58(1):41–7.

13. Moore ZS, Jerris RC, Hilinski JA. High prevalence of inducible clindamycin resis-tance among *Staphylococcus aureus* isolates from patients with cystic fibrosis. J Cyst Fibros 2008;7:206–9.

14. Yamaoka T. The bactericidal effects of anti-MRSA agents with rifampicin and sul-famethoxazole-trimethoprim against intracellular phagocytized MRSA. J Infect Chemother 2007;13(3):141–6.

15. Marangon FB, Miller D, Muallem MS, et al. Ciprofloxacin and levofloxacin resis-tance among methicillin-sensitive *Staphylococcus aureus* isolates from keratitis and conjunctivitis. Am J Ophthalmol 2004;137(3):453–8.

16. Horii T, Suzuki Y, Monji A, et al. Detection of mutations in quinolone resistance-determining regions in levofloxacin- and methicillin-resistant *Staphylococcus aureus*: effects of the mutations on fluoroquinolone MICs. Diagn Microbiol Infect Dis 2003;46(2):139–45.

17. Stein GE, Schooley S, Peloquin CA, et al. Linezolid tissue penetration and serum activity against strains of methicillin-resistant *Staphylococcus aureus* with reduced vancomycin susceptibility in diabetic patients with foot infections. J Anti-microb Chemother 2007;60:819–23.

18. Machado AR, Arns Cda C, Follador W, et al. Cost-effectiveness of linezolid versus vancomycin in mechanical ventilation-associated nosocomial pneumonia caused by methicillin-resistant *Staphylococcus aureus*. Braz J Infect Dis 2005;9(3): 191–200.

19. Weigelt J, Itani K, Stevens D, et al. Linezolid CSSTI Study Group. Linezolid versus vancomycin in treatment of complicated skin and soft tissue infections. Antimicrob Agents Chemother 2005;49(6):2260–6.

20. Sharpe JN, Shively EH, Polk HC Jr. Clinical and economic outcomes of oral linezolid versus intravenous vancomycin in the treatment of MRSA-complicated, lower-extremity skin and soft-tissue infections caused by methicillin-resistant *Staphylococcus aureus*. Am J Surg 2005;189(4):425–8.

21. Li JZ, Willke RJ, Rittenhouse BE, et al. Effect of linezolid versus vancomycin on length of hospital stay in patients with complicated skin and soft tissue infections caused by known or suspected methicillin-resistant Staphylococci: results from a randomized clinical trial. Surg Infect (Larchmt) 2003;4(1):57–70.

22. Lin DF, Zhang YY, Wu JF, et al. Linezolid for the treatment of infections caused by gram-positive pathogens in China. Int J Antimicrob Agents 2008;32:241–9.

23. Cunha BA. Methicillin-resistant *Staphylococcus aureus*: clinical manifestations and antimicrobial therapy. Clin Microbiol Infect 2005;11(Suppl 4):33–42.

24. Tally FP, Zeckel M, Wasilewski MM, et al. Daptomycin: a novel agent for Gram-positive infections. Expert Opin Investig Drugs 1999;8(8):1223–38.

25. Hsueh PR, Chen WH, Teng LJ, et al. Nosocomial infections due to methicillin-resistant *Staphylococcus aureus* and vancomycin-resistant Enterococci at a university hospital in Taiwan from 1991 to 2003: resistance trends, antibiotic usage and in vitro activities of newer antimicrobial agents. Int J Antimicrob Agents 2005;26(1):43–9.

26. LaPlante KL, Rybak MJ. Daptomycin – a novel antibiotic against Gram-positive pathogens. Expert Opin Pharmacother 2004;5(11):2321–31.

27. Bennett JW, Murray CK, Holmes RL, et al. Diminished vancomycin and daptomycin susceptibility during prolonged bacteremia with methicillin-resistant *Staphylococcus aureus*. Diagn Microbiol Infect Dis 2008;60(4):437–40.

28. Mangili A, Bica I, Snydman DR, et al. Daptomycin-resistant, methicillin-resistant *Staphylococcus aureus* bacteremia. Clin Infect Dis 2005;40(7):1058–60.

29. Hayden MK, Rezai K, Hayes RA, et al. Development of daptomycin resistance in vivo in methicillin-resistant *Staphylococcus aureus*. J Clin Microbiol 2005;43(10):5285–7.

30. Fritsche TR, Sader HS, Stilwell MG, et al. Potency and spectrum of tigecycline tested against an international collection of bacterial pathogens associated with skin and soft tissue infections (2000–2004). Diagn Microbiol Infect Dis 2005;52(3):195–201.

31. Bosó-Ribelles V, Romá-Sánchez E, Carmena J, et al. Tigecycline: a new treatment choice against *Acinetobacter baumannii*. Recent Pat AntiInfect Drug Discov 2008;3(2):117–22.

32. Luh KT, Hsueh PR, Teng LJ, et al. Quinupristin-dalfopristin resistance among gram-positive bacteria in Taiwan. Antimicrob Agents Chemother 2000;44(12):3374–80.

33. Saravolatz LD, Pawlak J, Johnson LB. Comparative activity of telavancin against isolates of community-associated methicillin-resistant *Staphylococcus aureus*. J Antimicrob Chemother 2007;60(2):406–9.

34. Jauregui LE, Babazadeh S, Seltzer E, et al. Randomized, double-blind comparison of once-weekly dalbavancin versus twice-daily linezolid therapy for the treatment of complicated skin and skin structure infections. Clin Infect Dis 2005;41(10):1407–15.

35. Imamura H, Ohtake N, Jona H, et al. Dicationic dithiocarbamate carbapenems with anti-MRSA activity. Bioorg Med Chem 2001;9(6):1571–8.

36. Kobayashi Y. Study of the synergism between carbapenems and vancomycin or teicoplanin against MRSA, focusing on S-4661, a carbapenem newly developed in Japan. J Infect Chemother 2005;11(5):259–61.
37. Bogdanovich T, Ednie LM, Shapiro S, et al. Antistaphylococcal activity of ceftobiprole, a new broad-spectrum cephalosporin. Antimicrob Agents Chemother 2005;49(10):4210–9.
38. Vaudaux P, Gjinovci A, Bento M, et al. Intensive therapy with ceftobiprole medocaril of experimental foreign-body infection by methicillin-resistant *Staphylococcus aureus*. Antimicrob Agents Chemother 2005;49(9):3789–93.
39. von Eiff C, Friedrich AW, Becker K, et al. Comparative in vitro activity of ceftobiprole against staphylococci displaying normal and small-colony variant phenotypes. Antimicrob Agents Chemother 2005;49(10):4372–4.
40. Lee CC, Tong KL, Howe HS, et al. *Vibrio vulnificus* infections: case reports and literature review. Ann Acad Med Singap 1997;26(5):705–12.
41. Jain R, Danziger LH. Multidrug-resistant Acinetobacter infections: an emerging challenge to clinicians. Ann Pharmacother 2004;38(9):1449–59.
42. Okubo H, Iwamoto M, Yoshio T, et al. Rapidly aggravated *Mycobacterium avium* infection in a patient with rheumatoid arthritis treated with infliximab. Mod Rheumatol 2005;15(1):62–4.
43. Rallis E, Koumantaki-Mathioudaki E, Frangoulis E, et al. Severe sporotrichoid fish tank granuloma following infliximab therapy. Am J Clin Dermatol 2007;8(6):385–8.
44. Salvana EM, Cooper GS, Salata RA. Mycobacterium other than tuberculosis (MOTT) infection: an emerging disease in infliximab-treated patients. J Infect 2007;55(6):484–7.
45. Sañudo A, Vallejo F, Sierra M, et al. Nontuberculous mycobacteria infection after mesotherapy: preliminary report of 15 cases. Int J Dermatol 2007;46(6):649–53.
46. Redbord KP, Shearer DA, Gloster H, et al. Atypical *Mycobacterium furunculosis* occurring after pedicures. J Am Acad Dermatol 2006;54(3):520–4.
47. Vugia DJ, Jang Y, Zizek C, et al. Mycobacteria in nail salon whirlpool footbaths, California. Emerg Infect Dis 2005;11(4):616–8.
48. Cooksey RC, de Waard JH, Yakrus MA, et al. *Mycobacterium cosmeticum* sp. nov., a novel rapidly growing species isolated from a cosmetic infection and from a nail salon. Int J Syst Evol Microbiol 2004;54(Pt 6):2385–91.
49. Gira AK, Reisenauer AH, Hammock L, et al. Furunculosis due to *Mycobacterium mageritense* associated with footbaths at a nail salon. J Clin Microbiol 2004;42(4):1813–7.
50. Giannella M, Pistella E, Perciaccante A, et al. Soft tissue infection caused by *Mycobacterium chelonae* following a liposculpture and lipofilling procedure. Ann Ital Med Int 2005;20(4):245–7.
51. Chetchotisakd P, Kiertiburanakul S, Mootsikapun P, et al. Disseminated nontuberculous mycobacterial infection in patients who are not infected with HIV in Thailand. Clin Infect Dis 2007;45(4):421–7.
52. Gomez MP, Herrera-Leon L, Jimenez MS, et al. Comparison of GenoType MTBC with RFLP-PCR and multiplex PCR to identify *Mycobacterium tuberculosis* complex species. Eur J Clin Microbiol Infect Dis 2007;26:63–6.
53. Kobashi Y, Obase Y, Fukuda M, et al. Clinical reevaluation of the QuantiFERON TB-2G test as a diagnostic method for differentiating active tuberculosis from nontuberculous mycobacteriosis. Clin Infect Dis 2006;43(12):1540–6.
54. Dodiuk-Gad R, Dyachenko P, Ziv M, et al. Nontuberculous mycobacterial infections of the skin: a retrospective study of 25 cases. J Am Acad Dermatol 2007;57(3):413–20.

55. Petrini B. *Mycobacterium marinum*: ubiquitous agent of waterborne granulomatous skin infections. Eur J Clin Microbiol Infect Dis 2006;25:609–13.

56. Fabroni C, Buggiani G, Lotti T. Therapy of environmental mycobacterial infections. Dermatol Ther 2008;21(3):162–6.

57. Cummins DL, Delacerda D, Tausk FA. *Mycobacterium marinum* with different responses to second-generation tetracyclines. Int J Dermatol 2005;44(6):518–20.

58. Petrini B. *Mycobacterium abscessus*: an emerging rapid-growing potential pathogen. APMIS 2006;114(5):319–28.

59. Musa MO, Al Eisa A, Halim M, et al. The spectrum of Fusarium infection in immunocompromised patients with haematological malignancies and in non-immunocompromised patients: a single institution experience over 10 years. Br J Haematol 2000;108(3):544–8.

60. Anaissie E, Kantarjian H, Ro J, et al. The emerging role of Fusarium infections in patients with cancer. Medicine (Baltimore) 1988;67(2):77–83.

61. Martino P, Gastaldi R, Raccah R, et al. Clinical patterns of Fusarium infections in immunocompromised patients. J Infect 1994;28(Suppl 1):7–15.

62. Cooper CR Jr, McGinnis MR. Pathology of *Penicillium marneffei*. An emerging acquired immunodeficiency syndrome-related pathogen. Arch Pathol Lab Med 1997;121(8):798–804.

63. Adler A, Yaniv I, Samra Z, et al. Exserohilum: an emerging human pathogen. Eur J Clin Microbiol Infect Dis 2006;25(4):247–53.

64. Ligon BL. Monkeypox: a review of the history and emergence in the Western hemisphere. Semin Pediatr Infect Dis 2004;15(4):280–7.

65. Kaur P, Ponniah M, Murhekar MV, et al. Chikungunya outbreak, South India, 2006. Emerg Infect Dis 2008;14(10):1623–5.

66. Mishra K, Rajawat V. Chikungunya-induced genital ulcers. Indian J Dermatol Venereol Leprol 2008;74(4):383–4.

67. Economopoulou A, Dominguez M, Helynck B, et al. Atypical chikungunya virus infections: clinical manifestations, mortality and risk factors for severe disease during the 2005–2006 outbreak on Réunion. Epidemiol Infect 2009;137(4):534–41.

Evaluation and Management of Psoriasis: An Internist's Guide

Danielle Levine, BA[a,b], Alice Gottlieb, MD, PhD[a,*]

KEYWORDS

- Psoriasis • Plaque • Immunopathogenesis • Biologics
- Metabolic syndrome

Psoriasis is a frustrating and often debilitating inflammatory skin disease that affects 0.6% to 4.8% of people worldwide.[1] Classically characterized by discrete erythematous plaques covered by a silvery white scale in characteristic locations, psoriasis may also present with pustular, guttate, and erythrodermic variants that share different features from the classic form. Patients who have psoriasis may initially present to their primary care office with no diagnosis but concerned about the cosmetic changes of their psoriatic lesions and the itching and pain often associated with these lesions.

Although the underlying cause of psoriasis is incompletely understood, recent evidence has linked psoriasis with atherosclerotic cardiovascular disease and the metabolic syndrome.[2] The relatively high prevalence of psoriasis mandates that primary care physicians be able to manage localized or mild disease and also be knowledgeable about treatment of moderate and severe disease to ensure appropriate dermatologic collaboration.

Disclosures: Neither manuscript nor any other related manuscripts have been published or submitted.

Alice Gottlieb, MD, PhD (as of November 1, 2008): Almost all income paid to employer directly. **Speakers' Bureau Memberships:** Amgen Inc; Wyeth Pharmaceuticals. **Current Consulting/Advisory Board Agreements:** Amgen Inc; Centocor, Inc; Wyeth Pharmaceuticals; Celgene Corp; Bristol Myers Squibb Co; Beiersdorf, Inc; Warner Chilcott; Abbott Laboratories; Roche; Sankyo; Medarex; Kemia; Celera; TEVA; Actelion; UCB; Novo Nordisk; Almirall; Immune Control; RxClinical; Dermipsor Ltd; Medacorp; DermiPsor; Can-Fite; Incyte; Pure-Tech; Magen Biosciences. **Research/Educational Grants:** Centocor; Amgen; Wyeth; Immune Control; Celgene; Pharmacare; Incyte; Abbott Laboratories; Pfizer (pending); Novo Nordisk (pending).

[a] Department of Dermatology, Tufts Medical Center, Tufts University School of Medicine, 800 Washington Street, Box #114, Boston, MA 02111, USA

[b] Department of Dermatology, Tufts Medical Center, Tufts University School of Medicine, 20 Stedman Street, Box #1, Boston, MA 02446, USA

* Corresponding author.

E-mail address: agottlieb@tuftsmedicalcenter.org (A. Gottlieb).

Med Clin N Am 93 (2009) 1291–1303

doi:10.1016/j.mcna.2009.08.003

0025-7125/09/$ – see front matter © 2009 Elsevier Inc. All rights reserved.

EPIDEMIOLOGY

Psoriasis is ubiquitous throughout the world.[1] It affects approximately 2.5% of the Caucasian population and 1.3% of the African American population in the United States, with approximately 150,000 newly diagnosed cases every year. The incidence of psoriasis is somewhat lower in Asians (0.4%).[3] Generally, it is more common in individuals living at higher latitudes or in colder locales, and less common in individuals who have greater sun exposure.

Psoriasis is equally common in men and women. It usually presents itself in a bimodal age distribution, with the earlier peak incidence between 15 and 30 years of age, and the later peak incidence between 50 and 60 years of age. The earlier peak is associated with more severe disease. This bimodal presentation has led to the definition of two forms of psoriasis: type I, often HLA-Cw6–associated, with age of onset before 40 years; and type II, which is not HLA-associated, with age of onset after 40 years. No current evidence shows that type I and type II psoriasis respond differently to different therapies.[4]

GENETICS AND RISK FACTORS

Genetic and environmental factors have been shown to predispose individuals to developing psoriasis. Based on population studies, the risk for psoriasis in children is estimated to be 41% if both parents are affected, 14% if one parent is affected, and 6% if one sibling is affected. Similarly, a family history can be found in 5% to 10% of patients who have psoriasis.[5] Recent evidence from HLA studies suggests a polygenic mode of inheritance, with certain class I major histocompatibility complex (MHC) antigens, particularly B13, B17, B39, and Cw6, and the class II MHC antigen DR7 occurring with increased frequency in relatives of patients who have psoriasis. The HLA antigens B27 and B38 are also associated with psoriatic arthritis.

In some families, variation at a single non-HLA genetic locus on chromosome 17q is linked to psoriasis susceptibility.[6] In other more recent studies, the *psoriasis susceptibility 1* locus, which is located in the MHC on chromosome 6p and is linked to the aforementioned HLA antigens, has been estimated to account for only one third to one half of the variation in genetic liability to psoriasis, suggesting that additional non-MHC genes are involved.[7]

As would be expected in a genetic disease, a higher concordance for psoriasis is seen in monozygotic versus dizygotic twins. However, the reported concordance for monozygotic twins has ranged from 35% to 73% in different studies, variability that points to nongenetic influences also playing a role in the pathogenesis of psoriasis.[8] Accordingly, several environmental triggers have been identified. Patients living in colder climates are at greater risk for developing the disease, probably because they are exposed to less ultraviolet radiation, which has been shown to be protective against psoriatic lesions (see later discussion on phototherapy). Smoking is associated with an increased risk for psoriasis and increased severity of the disease.[9] Psoriasis may also be exacerbated by streptococcal infection and certain drugs, particularly interferon-α, lithium, antimalarials, abrupt cessation of systemic corticosteroids, and β-blockers. Psoriasis can also be the presenting sign of HIV infection, and HIV-associated psoriasis is classically more severe than the common form. An association has also been seen between psoriasis and obesity and alcohol consumption, but whether these factors may actually cause the disease or are a result of having psoriasis is unclear.[10]

The *Koebner phenomenon*, also known as the isomorphic response, is the occurrence of psoriasis in areas of trauma. It usually occurs 1 to 2 weeks after injury in an all-or-none pattern, with psoriatic lesions appearing at either all or no sites of injury. Approximately 25% of patients report a history of the Koebner phenomenon at some point in their lives, and estimates of lifetime prevalence rise as high as 76% when coupled with infection and stress.[4]

CLINICAL MANIFESTATIONS AND DIAGNOSIS

Psoriasis is diagnosed through physical examination. Psoriasis usually presents with symmetric, well-demarcated, erythematous plaques with overlying silvery scales, often with accompanying pruritus (**Fig. 1**A–D). Single lesions may become confluent, extend laterally, or develop partial central clearing. Removing the silvery scales induces trauma to the underlying dilated capillaries and results in pinpoint bleeding in the site of the lesion, a finding known as the *Auspitz sign*. Although psoriasis may affect almost any part of the body, it most commonly appears on the elbows, knees, scalp, gluteal cleft, umbilicus, and lower back. The Koebner phenomenon may explain why the knees and elbows are common sites for psoriatic lesions, because chronic trauma is often experienced in these regions. Nail involvement, particularly pitting, onycholysis, and red-brown discoloration resembling drops of oil, more often in fingers than toes, can occur in up to 50% of patients. Geographic tongue, which presents as asymptomatic erythematous patches on the tongue correlating with loss of filiform papillae, may also be seen, although it is nonspecific. A seronegative inflammatory arthritis is seen in approximately 25% of patients, and these patients who have *psoriatic arthritis* (PsA) are more likely to also have nail abnormalities. In PsA, skin disease usually precedes joint disease by an average of 12 years in 84% of patients (**Fig. 1**F).[11]

This pattern of psoriasis represents the most common form of the disease—plaque-type psoriasis or psoriasis vulgaris—seen in approximately 90% of patients. Approximately one third of patients who have psoriasis vulgaris are reported to have moderate-to-severe disease based on their extensively involved body surface area or the significant impact on their quality of life.[12]

In addition to psoriasis vulgaris, the disease has four other variants: guttate, inverse, pustular, and erythrodermic. Guttate ("drop-like") psoriasis, which is most associated with HLA-Cw6,[4] consists of numerous 0.5- to 1.5-cm papules over the trunk and proximal extremities, and often erupts suddenly. Inverse psoriasis is characterized by sharply demarcated erythema without scale, localized to intertriginous areas such as the axillae, genital folds, or neck. Inverse psoriasis must therefore be distinguished from fungal infections.

The pustular and erythrodermic psoriatic variants are potentially more severe and life-threatening. In pustular psoriasis, pustules develop either in a rim around plaques, on the palmoplantar surfaces, or throughout the body. The latter form may be accompanied by high fevers, leukocytosis, and hepatotoxicity, and often requires inpatient systemic therapy. Similar widespread involvement is observed in the erythrodermic psoriatic variant, characterized by generalized erythema and scaling from head to toe (**Fig. 1**E). These patients, like those who have sustained burns, are at increased risk for infection, severe dehydration, and electrolyte loss and must also be treated aggressively in the inpatient setting.[13]

Once the diagnosis of psoriasis is suggested through physical examination, a careful history is important in defining the nature of the disease and determining appropriate treatment. Physicians should document the age of onset, family history, and prior course of the disease. Of important prognostic implication is the history of relapse, because patients who frequently experience relapse tend to develop more severe

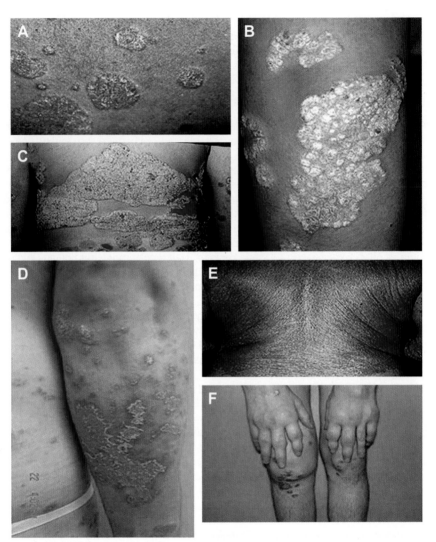

Fig. 1. Patients who have (*A*) small plaque psoriasis, (*B*) localized thick plaque-type psoriasis, (*C*) large plaque psoriasis, (*D*) inflammatory localized psoriasis, (*E*) erythrodermic psoriasis, and (*F*) psoriasis and psoriatic arthritis. (*From* Menter A, Gottlieb A, Feldman SR, et al. Guidelines of care for the management of psoriasis and psoriatic arthritis: Section 1. Overview of psoriasis and guidelines of care for the treatment of psoriasis with biologics. J Am Acad Dermatol 2008;58(5):826–50; with permission.)

disease, with rapidly enlarging lesions covering significant parts of the body, and may require more aggressive therapy. Physicians should also inquire about current medications, joint complaints, and previous response to therapy.

Psoriatic plaques may occasionally resemble atopic dermatitis, or eczema, but will usually be thicker, redder, and more sharply demarcated than eczematous lesions. Furthermore, psoriasis usually affects the extensor surfaces on the knees and elbows, whereas eczema typically involved the flexor surfaces. Psoriatic plaques may occasionally resemble seborrheic dermatitis, tinea infections, cutaneous T-cell lymphoma, ichthyosis, secondary syphilis, and Reiter's syndrome.[11] In the few cases in which physical examination and clinical history are not diagnostic, skin biopsy may be indicated to make the diagnosis. Classic histopathologic features of psoriasis include epidermal hyperplasia with parakeratosis (retention of nuclei in the stratum corneum), a neutrophil-rich stratum corneum (Munro's abscess), thinning of the granular layer of the epidermis, and a mononuclear dermal and epidermal infiltrate. Infiltration of T cells and dendritic cells in plaques and dysregulated angiogenesis of dermal blood vessels[14] have also been described (**Fig. 2**).

PATHOGENESIS

Psoriatic immunopathogenesis consists of the complex interplay among innate and acquired immune cell types and among immune factors produced by dendritic cells, T cells, and keratinocytes in the psoriatic plaque.[15] Effector cells of innate immunity in psoriatic lesions include neutrophils and dendritic cells. In psoriatic lesions and arthritic joints, dendritic cells express tumor necrosis factor α (TNFα), an inflammatory cytokine that up-regulates nuclear factor-κB (NF-κB) and can thereby induce inflammatory molecules such as interleukin (IL)-1, IL-8, IL-6, and inducible nitric oxide synthase (iNOS). iNOS, in turn, may facilitate nitric oxide production, thereby causing capillary vasodilatation.[16–23] TNFα could also promote emigration of leukocytes into the skin, induce adhesion molecule expression, and up-regulate vascular endothelial growth factor (VEGF), further facilitating inflammation and angiogenesis in the psoriatic plaque.

In addition to expressing TNFα, dendritic cells produce the cytokine IL-23. IL-23 is known to be a critical player in psoriatic immunopathogenesis through its effects on Th17 T-cell development and production of cytokines such as IL-17 and IL-22.

COMORBIDITIES

Although primarily a disease of the skin, psoriasis is now known to be inextricably linked to several other diseases. Recent evidence has even suggested an increased overall risk for mortality with a hazard ratio of 1.5 (95% CI, 1.3–1.7) in especially young patients who have severe psoriasis.[24] An average of 25% of patients who have psoriasis also develop the inflammatory seronegative spondyloarthropathy PsA, characterized by stiffness, pain, swelling, and tenderness of the joints and surrounding ligaments and tendons (dactylitis and enthesitis). In addition to digital involvement, enthesitis in PsA commonly involves insertion sites of the plantar fascia, the Achilles' tendons, and ligamentous attachments to the ribs, spine, and pelvis. Nail disease is frequently seen in PsA, especially in patients who have distal interphalangeal (DIP) joint involvement. If untreated, PsA can develop into debilitating, erosive arthropathy characterized by persistent inflammation, progressive joint damage, physical disability, and increased mortality.[25]

In addition to their risk for developing PsA, patients who have psoriasis are believed to have a genetic susceptibility to autoimmune disease and dysregulation of TNFα, and therefore are more likely to develop Crohn's disease than individuals who do not have psoriasis.[26] Psoriasis has also been shown to occur more commonly in families of patients who have multiple sclerosis compared with controls,[27] although it is unclear whether patients who have psoriasis are at higher risk for developing multiple sclerosis.

Patients who have psoriasis also have an increased risk for metabolic syndrome and cardiovascular disease, suggesting that the chronic inflammation of psoriasis may be a risk factor for cardiometabolic pathology, perhaps for the same reason that

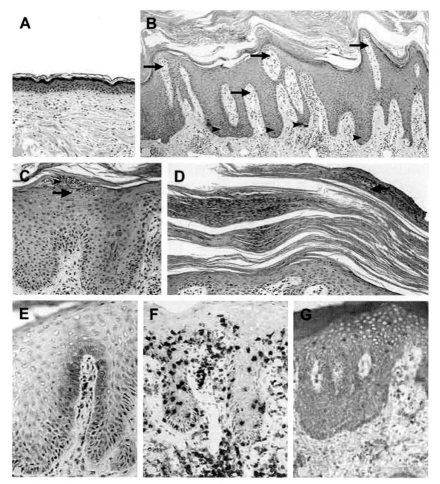

Fig. 2. Histopathologic changes in psoriatic skin. (*A*) normal skin. (*B*) Epidermis in psoriatic skin, characterized by acanthosis (thickening of the viable cell layers), elongation of epidermal rete ridges (*arrowheads*), hyperkeratosis (thickening of the cornified layer), loss of the granular layer, parakeratosis (nuclei in the stratum corneum), dilated dermal blood vessels that nearly reach the epidermis (*arrows*), and a mixed leukocytic infiltrate seen in both dermis and epidermis. (*C*) Neutrophilic granulocytes have transmigrated through the epidermis (*arrow*) and have formed a Munro microabscess underneath the stratum corneum (*arrowhead*). As the lesions progress, these microabscesses are transported to the upper layers of the stratum corneum, where they slough off (*D, arrow*). Focal expression of epidermal intercellular adhesion molecule 1 (ICAM-1) indicates keratinocyte activation (*E*), and immunostaining of CD3 (a T-cell receptor–associated antigen) indicates the abundance of T cells within dermis and epidermis (*F*). In addition, immunostaining of the $_E$(CD103)$_7$ integrin, an adhesion receptor that binds to epidermal E-cadherin, reveals almost exclusive expression by intraepidermal T cells (*G*). ICAM-1 and the $_E$(CD103)$_7$ integrin contribute to the recruitment of pathogenic lymphocytes to psoriatic skin. (*From* Schön MP, Boehncke WH. Psoriasis. N Engl J Med 2005;352:1899–912; with permission.)

C-reactive protein is used as a biomarker for coronary disease. In a hospital-based case-control study on 338 adult patients who had chronic plaque psoriasis, Gisondi and colleagues[28] observed that the metabolic syndrome was significantly more common in patients who had psoriasis than in controls (30.1% versus. 20.6%; odds ratio, 1.65; P<.005) after the age of 40 years, independent of the incidence of smoking. This association showed a time-course relationship, with patients experiencing psoriasis for the longest time also having the highest prevalence of metabolic syndrome. In this study, patients who had psoriasis also had a higher prevalence of hypertriglyceridemia and abdominal obesity.

Similarly, evidence from the United Kingdom General Practice Database, which contains data on more than 130,000 patients who have psoriasis aged 20 to 90 years, has shown that patients who have psoriasis have a higher-than-normal incidence of myocardial infarction, even after correcting for classic atherosclerotic risk factors, such as smoking, diabetes, obesity, hypertension, and hyperlipidemia.[29,30] To what extent immunobiologic and other anti-inflammatory therapies may also reduce the risk for cardiovascular disease in patients who have psoriasis remains to be determined.

Some evidence shows that patients who have psoriasis have an increased lifetime risk for also developing lymphoma. In a retrospective cohort study of 2718 patients who had psoriasis in the United Kingdom, Gelfand and colleagues[31] found that patients who had psoriasis had a 2.95 relative rate of developing lymphoma compared with the general population, independent of age, gender, and methotrexate therapy.

In addition to their higher risk for developing medical comorbidities, patients who have psoriasis are more prone to mood disorders, including depression, which occurs in as many as 60% of patients, and a substantial proportion of these patients may actively contemplate suicide.[30] Importantly, a recent multicenter randomized phase III trial comparing twice-weekly etanercept therapy with placebo in more than 600 adults who had moderate-to-severe plaque psoriasis found that patients treated with etanercept had a significant decrease in their Hamilton rating scale for depression scores (suggesting that they had fewer symptoms of depression) compared with control subjects.[32]

TREATMENT

Patients who have psoriasis report an impaired quality of life to a degree that rivals that caused by other major illnesses such as diabetes and cancer.[33] At the same time, treatment of the disease presents many challenges for patients and health care providers. The goal of treatment is long-term, safe, and effective clearance of psoriatic lesions. Part of the challenge in treating psoriasis is that traditional psoriatic treatments are only somewhat effective (eg, topical agents), inconvenient (eg, phototherapy), or toxic (eg, methotrexate); these attributes lead to poor patient compliance and increase the tendency for psoriatic flares.

Over the past 10 years, targeted immunobiologic therapies have been and are being developed aimed at creating the ideal therapy to clear psoriasis and that can be safely and effectively used on a chronic basis.[25] These therapies, which incorporate current understanding of psoriatic immunopathogenesis, are rapidly transforming the management of moderate-to-severe psoriasis for patients and providers alike. This section focuses on treatment of patients who have psoriasis; discussion of PsA therapy is beyond the scope of this review.

Current treatments for psoriasis can be compartmentalized into five categories: topical applications, phototherapy, traditional systemic treatments, immunobiologics, and experimental approaches. As with many diseases that can present with increasing degrees of severity, treatment modalities for psoriasis are selected based on extent of disease, patient preference, comorbidities, and individual patient response. The traditional approach to treatment of psoriasis categorizes patients into two groups. The first group, which encompasses 75% of patients and includes individuals who have mild or localized disease that does not significantly impact quality of life, are generally managed with topical therapy as the first line of treatment.[34] The second traditional treatment group includes the remaining 25% of patients who have moderate-to-severe psoriasis that affects quality of life, and these patients often require more aggressive systemic therapy. Of course, even in the first group, location of lesions (eg, genitals or face), previous failure of topical therapy, excessive inconvenience, history of frequent relapsing disease, or presence of psoriatic arthritis may also prompt the consideration of systemic therapy.

Topical therapies include emollients, corticosteroids, vitamin D analogs, the vitamin A analog tazarotene, topical immunosuppressants, tars, and anthralin. Emollients are important to maintain skin hydration, minimize itching, and avoid Koebnerization.[35] Topical corticosteroids are at once anti-inflammatory, antiproliferative, and immunosuppressive and are the mainstay of topical psoriatic therapy because of their short-term efficacy and broad range of potency. In choosing a topical corticosteroid, physicians must consider the anatomic site, thickness of the psoriatic plaque, extent of involvement, and relative contraindications (eg, preexisting skin atrophy). Although the typical corticosteroid regimen consists typically of twice-daily topical applications, some regimens that involve especially potent corticosteroid preparations recommend infrequent applications (eg, every weekend), a schedule known as pulse therapy.[19]

The vitamin D analogs, calcipotriene and tacalcitol, and the vitamin A analog tazarotene, are somewhat affective in reversing keratinocyte hyperproliferation and thereby reducing the severity of psoriatic plaques. Several recent trials found that combined use of daily calcipotriene and superpotent corticosteroids, either halobetasol in a pulse therapy pattern or daily betamethasone, may actually be more efficacious and better tolerated than either agent alone.[36,37] The calcineurin inhibitors tacrolimus and pimecrolimus have been studied as steroid-sparing agents in patients who have plaque psoriasis, but a recent FDA warning linking these medications with certain types of lymphoma has curtailed their use of late.[35] Keratolytics are used to decrease scale. Finally, topical coal tar preparations and anthralin are traditional modalities that have been historically tedious to use; these therapies have largely fallen out of favor by the medical community in light of the newer corticosteroid and vitamin D analog preparations.

Patients who have more sun exposure have a lower risk for developing psoriasis because of the antiproliferative and anti-inflammatory effects of ultraviolet light on psoriatic plaques. Therefore, phototherapy with ultraviolet B (UVB) radiation and the more potent photochemotherapy with psoralen plus ultraviolet A radiation (PUVA) are still occasionally used in patients who have moderate-to-severe psoriasis. PUVA penetrates deeper into the dermis and is usually used when UVB fails. However, because of the highly technical nature of these treatment modalities, and because several recent studies have highlighted a worrisome link between prolonged PUVA phototherapy and squamous cell carcinoma and melanoma,[38] these treatments should be reserved for specially trained dermatologists.

When psoriasis is moderate-to-severe, the physician should consider systemic therapy. Specific indications for systemic therapy include moderate-to-severe plaque psoriasis, usually involving at least 10% of the body surface area; failure of topical treatment; incapacitating disease affecting quality of life; PsA; or generalized pustular or erythrodermic psoriasis. Traditional therapies in this category include methotrexate (MTX), cyclosporine, and acitretin.

In addition to preventing epidermal hyperproliferation by inhibiting dihydrofolate reductase (DHFR), MTX is believed to prevent the proliferation of T cells by also inhibiting aminoimidazole carboxamide ribonucleotide, an enzyme involved in purine metabolism.[4] It is administered orally, intramuscularly, or subcutaneously, usually in once-weekly (7.5–25 mg) regimens. Although effective, MTX has many side effects, including hepatotoxicity, bone marrow suppression, pneumonitis, abortion, and teratogenicity. These side effects can be observed even with concomitant administration of folic acid. As a result of the potential for hepatotoxicity, prior guidelines suggest a liver biopsy after a 1.5-g cumulative dose.[39]

Cyclosporine (CsA) is another immunosuppressive medication that works rapidly and is effective in most patients.[30] In psoriasis, CsA inhibits keratinocyte hyperproliferation and prevents production of IL-2, thereby impairing helper T-cell activation. In a large randomized control trial published in 1991, Ellis and colleagues[40] found that 8 weeks of CsA dose-dependently cleared the plaques of patients who had moderate-to-severe psoriasis, compared with no clearance of plaques in patients treated with placebo. At the same time, significant side effects can be observed, including nephrotoxicity, hypertension, hypercholesterolemia, increased infection, hirsutism, gum hypertrophy, headache and tremor, and a potential increase in cutaneous and internal malignancies.

The final FDA-approved traditional systemic therapy for psoriasis is acitretin, a systemic retinoid indicated for patients who have severe plaque psoriasis and for pustular and erythrodermic forms of the disease. When used to treat severe plaque psoriasis, acitretin is often combined with UVB or PUVA phototherapy as a dose-sparing approach.[41] However, acitretin is teratogenic, and has been associated with mucocutaneous side effects, hypertriglyceridemia, and hepatotoxicity.

Recent advances in understanding the immunopathogenesis of psoriasis has led to the development of a promising class of immunomodulatory medications known as *biologics*. The biologics are recombinant proteins (either monoclonal antibodies or fusion proteins) extracted from animal tissue that target activated T cells, adhesion molecules, or chemokines that play a role in psoriasis.[42] These medications are revolutionizing the management of psoriasis because they are highly effective and well tolerated by patients. In clinical trials, medication efficacy is recorded with the Psoriasis Area and Severity Index (PASI) score, a measure of overall psoriasis severity and coverage that assesses body surface area and erythema, induration, and scaling. A 75% improvement in the PASI score (PASI-75) is usually used to document the effectiveness of specific therapies in clinical trials. Some trials used the Physicians Global Assessment (PGA), which requires the investigator to assign a single estimate of the patient's overall severity of disease on a 5- to 6-point scale.

Five biologic agents are currently approved by the FDA: alefacept (Amevive) and efalizumab (Raptiva), which target pathogenic T cells, and adalimumab (Humira), etanercept (Enbrel), and infliximab (Remicade), which target TNFα.[43] Newer agents are also currently being tested in clinical trials.

As a general rule, the National Psoriasis Foundation recommends that psoriasis patients taking biologics should be monitored with baseline and periodic blood work, including chemistry screen with liver function tests, complete blood count, hepatitis panel, and tuberculosis testing. Specific medications may require additional monitoring based on side effect profiles. Because the biologics are immunosuppressive, patients on these medications and methotrexate and cyclosporine must avoid live attenuated vaccinations and must be carefully monitored for signs or symptoms of infection.[44]

The recombinant dimeric fusion protein alefacept binds to CD2 on memory effector T lymphocytes, thereby inhibiting the number of these cells in psoriatic plaques. It is FDA-approved as a 12-week, 15-mg intramuscular injection for the treatment of adult patients who have moderate-to-severe chronic plaque psoriasis who are candidates for systemic agents or phototherapy. Phase III trials showed that 21% of patients achieved a PASI75 score 2 weeks after the twelfth injection of alefacept.[43] A recent study found that patients may benefit from up to two additional 12-week therapeutic courses of alefacept, with the greatest clinical responses seen with concomitant UVB therapy.[45] Because of alefacept's inhibitory effect on T cells, patients taking this medication should have their CD4 counts checked before treatment and every other week on treatment.[46] Patients infected with HIV who have psoriasis are not candidates for alefacept therapy.

Efalizumab is a recombinant monoclonal antibody directed against the CD11a subunit of the integrin (LFA-1) responsible for T-cell adhesion. It is FDA-approved for adults who have chronic moderate-to-severe plaque psoriasis and is administered weekly as a subcutaneous injection: 0.7 mg/kg for the initiation dose followed by 1-mg/kg weekly doses thereafter.[30] In a phase III randomized, placebo-controlled, double-blind study of nearly 600 patients who had psoriasis treated with efalizumab or placebo, Lebwohl and colleagues[47] found that 22% of the patients treated with efalizumab, 1 mg/kg per week, and 28% of the patients treated with efalizumab, 2 mg/kg per week, had achieved PASI-75 at week 12, compared with only 5% of patients treated with placebo. A similar trend was observed at week 24 of efalizumab versus placebo treatment. Even after the discontinuation of efalizumab at week 24, in fact, an improvement of 50% or more in the PASI was maintained in approximately 30% of patients during 12 weeks of follow-up. Despite this encouraging data, efalizumab is not effective against PsA; it has also been associated with psoriatic arthritis flares during therapy, psoriasis rebound, flu-like symptoms, hemolytic anemia, thrombocytopenia, peripheral demyelination, and progressive multifocal leukoencephalopathy.[30]

The second group of FDA-approved biologics encompasses the TNF inhibitors, three of which are approved for use in both psoriasis and psoriatic arthritis. Adalimumab, a fully human anti-TNFα monoclonal antibody, is effective against moderate-to-severe plaque psoriasis and PsA, and also may be effective long-term. A recent 52-week, multicenter study of 1212 patients who had psoriasis randomized to either adalimumab or placebo every other week found that 71% of those treated with adalimumab achieved PASI-75 at week 16, compared with 7% of those treated with placebo. This study also observed that when the patients who had achieved PASI-75 after 33 weeks of continuous adalimumab therapy were re-randomized in a double-blind manner to either continued adalimumab or placebo, only 5% of those re-randomized to adalimumab lost adequate response (defined as <50% improvement in the PASI response relative to baseline and at least a six-point increase in PASI score from week 33), compared with 28% of patients re-randomized to placebo.[48] Adalimumab is currently approved for moderate to severe psoriasis treatment in a dosing regimen of 80 mg subcutaneously the first week, followed by 40 mg subcutaneously the next week and then every 2 weeks thereafter.

Etanercept, a recombinant human TNFα receptor protein fused with the Fc portion of IgG1, is FDA-approved when given in dosing regimens of 50 mg subcutaneously twice weekly for the first 12 weeks followed by 50 mg weekly thereafter for moderate-to-severe plaque psoriasis and for PsA. A randomized trial of etanercept in 652 adult patients who had plaque psoriasis noted an improvement from baseline of PASI-75 or more in 34% of the etanercept group receiving 25 mg twice weekly and 49% of the etanercept group receiving 50 mg twice weekly, compared with 4%

of the patients in the placebo group. In fact, the clinical responses continued to improve with 24-week treatment.[30,49] Etanercept is FDA-approved for treating moderate to severe psoriasis as follows: 50 mg subcutaneously twice weekly for 12 weeks followed by step-down to 50 mg once-weekly dosing.

Infliximab is a chimeric antibody that binds to and inhibits TNFα; it is now FDA-approved for severe psoriasis and PsA. In phase III trials, 75.5% to 80% of patients who had psoriasis experienced a PASI-75 response after induction therapy (5 mg/kg intravenous infusions at weeks 0, 2, and 6). After adding maintenance dosing of infliximab every 8 weeks through 46 weeks, 61% of patients had at least a 75% improvement at week 50.[23,43,50,51]

Because TNFα inhibitors have been used for nearly 10 years as part of the treatment armamentarium for rheumatoid arthritis and inflammatory bowel disease, the potential toxicities of these medications are now well understood. TNFα inhibitors carry the potential for increased risk for serious infections, including opportunistic infections; demyelinating disorders; hepatotoxicity; lupus-like syndromes; pancytopenias; lymphoma; and non-melanoma skin cancers.[30] However, TNFα inhibitors are usually given as monotherapy for psoriasis but are often prescribed alongside additional immunosuppressive therapy for rheumatoid arthritis and inflammatory bowel disease, so the side effects observed with TNFα inhibitor therapy for rheumatoid arthritis and inflammatory bowel disease may overestimate the expected side effects of TNFα inhibitor therapy for psoriasis.[30]

REFERENCES

1. Naldi L. Epidemiology of psoriasis. Curr Drug Targets Inflamm Allergy 2004;3: 121.
2. Gottlieb AB, Dann F, Menter A. Psoriasis and the metabolic syndrome. J Drugs Dermatol 2008;7(6):563–72.
3. Gelfand JM, Stern RS, Nijsten T, et al. The prevalence of psoriasis in African-Americans: results from a population-based study. J Am Acad Dermatol 2005; 52:23.
4. Gudjonsson JE, Elder JT. Psoriasis. In: Wolff K, Goldsmith LA, Katz SL, et al, editors. Fitzpatrick's dermatology in general medicine. 7th edition. New York: McGraw-Hill; 2008. p. 170–93.
5. Elder JT, Nair RP, Guo SW, et al. The genetics of psoriasis. Arch Dermatol 1994; 130:216.
6. Tomfohrde J, Silverman A, Barnes R, et al. Gene for familial psoriasis susceptibility mapped to the distal end of human chromosome 17q. Science 1994;264: 1141.
7. Sagoo GS, Cork MJ, Patel R, et al. Genome-wide studies of psoriasis susceptibility loci: a review. J Dermatol Sci 2004;35:171.
8. Huerta C, Rivero E, Rodríguez LA. Incidence and risk factors for psoriasis in the general population. Arch Dermatol 2007;143:1559.
9. Setty AR, Curhan G, Choi HK. Smoking and the risk of psoriasis in women: Nurses' Health Study II. Am J Med 2007;120:953.
10. Sterry W, Strober BE, Menter A. Obesity in psoriasis: the metabolic, clinical and therapeutic implications, report of an interdisciplinary conference and review. Br J Dermatol 2007;157:649–55.
11. Wenzel FG, Morison WL. Psoriasis. In: Stein JH, Sande MA, Zvaifler NA, et al, editors. Internal medicine. 5th edition. St Louis (MO): Mosby; 1998. p. 2041–50.
12. Gottlieb AB. Psoriasis. Dis Manag Clin Outcomes 1998;1:195–202.

13. Boyd AS, Menter A. Erythrodermic psoriasis. Precipitating factors, course, and prognosis in 50 patients. J Am Acad Dermatol 1989;21:985.

14. Ragaz A, Ackerman AB. Evolution, maturation, and regression of lesions of psoriasis. New observations and correlation of clinical and histologic findings. Am J Dermatopathol 1979;1(3):199–214.

15. Lowes MA, Bowcock AM, Krueger JG. Pathogenesis and therapy of psoriasis. Nature 2007;445(7130):866–73.

16. Gottlieb AB. Psoriasis: emerging therapeutic strategies. Nat Rev Drug Discov 2005;4(1):19–34.

17. Zhou X, Krueger JG, Kao MC, et al. Novel mechanisms of T-cell and dendritic cell activation revealed by profiling of psoriasis on the 63,100-element oligonucleotide array. Physiol Genomics 2003;13:69–78.

18. Bettelli E, Carrier Y, Gao W, et al. Reciprocal developmental pathways for the generation of pathogenic effector TH17 and regulatory T cells. Nature 2006; 441:235–8.

19. Lee E, Trepicchio WL, Oestreicher JL, et al. Increased expression if interleukin 23 p19 and p40 in lesional skin of patients with psoriasis vulgaris. J Exp Med 2004; 199:125–30.

20. Wilson NJ, Boniface K, Chan JR, et al. Development, cytokine profile and function of human interleukin 17–producing helper T cells. Nat Immunol 2007;8(9):950–7.

21. Asarch A, Barak O, Loo DS, et al. Th17 cells: a new paradigm for cutaneous inflammation. J Dermatolog Treat 2008;19(5):259–66.

22. Chan JR, Blumenschein W, Murphy E, et al. IL-23 stimulates epidermal hyperplasia via TNF and IL-20R2-dependent mechanisms with implications for psoriasis pathogenesis. J Exp Med 2006;203:2577–87.

23. Krueger GG, Langley RG, Leonardi C, et al. A human interleukin-12/23 monoclonal antibody for the treatment of psoriasis. N Engl J Med 2007;356:580–92.

24. Gelfand JM, Troxel AB, Lewis JD, et al. The risk of mortality in patients with psoriasis: results from a population-based study. Arch Dermatol 2007;143:1493–9.

25. Gottlieb A, Korman NJ, Gordon KB, et al. Guidelines of care for the management of psoriasis and psoriatic arthritis: section 2. Psoriatic arthritis: overview and guidelines of care for treatment with an emphasis on the biologics. J Am Acad Dermatol 2008;58(5):851–64.

26. Najarian DJ, Gottlieb AB. Connections between psoriasis and Crohn's disease. J Am Acad Dermatol 2003;48:805–21.

27. Broadley SA, Deans J, Sawcer SJ, et al. Autoimmune disease in first-degree relatives of patients with multiple sclerosis: a UK survey. Brain 2000;123:1102–11.

28. Gisondi P, Tessari G, Conti A, et al. Prevalence of metabolic syndrome in patients with psoriasis: a hospital-based case-control study. Br J Dermatol 2007;157:68–73.

29. Gelfand JM, Neimann AL, Shin DB, et al. Risk of myocardial infarction in patients with psoriasis. JAMA 2006;296:1735–41.

30. Menter A, Gottlieb A, Feldman SR, et al. Guidelines of care for the management of psoriasis and psoriatic arthritis: section 1. Overview of psoriasis and guidelines of care for the treatment of psoriasis with biologics. J Am Acad Dermatol 2008; 58(5):826–50.

31. Gelfand JM, Berlin J, Van Voorhees A, et al. Lymphoma rates are low but increased in patients with psoriasis: results from a population-based cohort study in the United Kingdom. Arch Dermatol 2003;139:1425–9.

32. Tyring S, Gottlieb A, Papp K, et al. Etanercept and clinical outcomes, fatigue, and depression in psoriasis: double-blind placebo-controlled randomized phase III trial. Lancet 2006;367:29–35.

33. Rapp SR, Feldman SR, Exum ML, et al. Psoriasis causes as much disability as other major medical diseases. J Am Acad Dermatol 1999;41:401–7.
34. Stern RS, Nijsten T, Feldman SR, et al. Psoriasis is common, carries a substantial burden even when not extensive, and is associated with widespread treatment dissatisfaction. J Investig Dermatol Symp Proc 2004;9:136–9.
35. Feldman SR, Pearce DJ. Treatment of psoriasis. In: Dellavalle section editor. UpToDate, version 16.2. May 2008. Available at: www.uptodate.com. Accessed October 23, 2008.
36. Koo J, Blum RR, Lebwohl M. A randomized, multicenter study of calcipotriene ointment and clobetasol propionate foam in the sequential treatment of localized plaque-type psoriasis: short- and long-term outcomes. J Am Acad Dermatol 2006;55:637.
37. Kaufmann R, Bibby AJ, Bissonnette R, et al. A new calcipotriol/betamethasone dipropionate formulation (Daivobet) is an effective once-daily treatment for psoriasis vulgaris. Dermatology 2002;205:389.
38. Stern RS. The risk of melanoma in association with long-term exposure to PUVA. J Am Acad Dermatol 2001;44:755.
39. Roenigk HH Jr, Auerbach R, Maibach HI, et al. Methotrexate in psoriasis: revised guidelines. J Am Acad Dermatol 1988;19:145–56.
40. Ellis CN, Fradin MS, Messana MD, et al. Cyclosporine for plaque-type psoriasis. Results of a multidose, double-blind trial. N Engl J Med 1991;324:277–84.
41. Lebwohl M, Drake L, Menter A, et al. Consensus conference: acitretin in combination with UVB or PUVA in the treatment of psoriasis. J Am Acad Dermatol 2001; 45:544.
42. Krueger JG. The immunologic basis for the treatment of psoriasis with new biologic agents. J Am Acad Dermatol 2002;46:1–23.
43. Berger EM, Gottlieb AB. Developments in systemic immunomodulatory therapy for psoriasis. Curr Opin Pharmacol 2007;7(4):434–44.
44. Lebwohl M, Bagel J, Gelfand JM, et al. From the medical board of the National Psoriasis Foundation: monitoring and vaccinations in patients treated with biologics for psoriasis. J Am Acad Dermatol 2008;58:94–105.
45. Krueger GG, Gottlieb AB, Sterry W, et al. A multicenter, open-label study of repeat courses of intramuscular alefacept in combination with other psoriasis therapies in patients with chronic plaque psoriasis. J Dermatolog Treat 2008; 19(3):146–55.
46. Alafecept. [package insert]. Available at. http://www.fda.gov/cder/foi/label/2003/alefbio013003LB.htm. Accessed November 22, 2008.
47. Lebwohl M, Tyring SK, Hamilton TK, et al. A novel targeted T-cell modulator, efalizumab, for plaque psoriasis. N Engl J Med 2003;349(21):2004–13.
48. Menter A, Tyring SK, Gordon K, et al. Adalimumab therapy for moderate to severe psoriasis: a randomized, controlled phase III trial. J Am Acad Dermatol 2007;58: 106–15.
49. Leonardi CL, Powers JL, Matheson RT, et al. Etanercept as monotherapy in patients with psoriasis. N Engl J Med 2003;349:2014–22.
50. Reich K, Nestle FO, Papp K. Infliximab induction and maintenance therapy for moderate-to-severe psoriasis: a phase III, multicentre, double-blind trial. Lancet 2005;366:1367–74.
51. Gottlieb AB, Evans R, Li S, et al. Infliximab induction therapy for patients with severe plaque-type psoriasis: a randomized, doubleblind, placebo-controlled trial. J Am Acad Dermatol 2004;51:534–42.

Facial Papules as a Marker of Internal Malignancy

Ravi Ubriani, MD*, Marc E. Grossman, MD

KEYWORDS

- Malignancy • Cutaneous • Marker • Facial • Papule

Facial papules (bumps) confront the general practitioner during every face-to-face meeting with the patient (**Tables 1** and **2**). Increased awareness and recognition of the facial papules that represent cutaneous signs of internal malignancy will allow an early, aggressive workup and treatment of any associated cancer. A skin biopsy for histopathologic diagnosis is necessary to distinguish these clues to underlying malignancy from the numerous benign lesions that cause facial papules.

SKIN-COLORED PAPULES
Birt-Hogg-Dubé Syndrome

Overview

Birt-Hogg-Dubé syndrome (BHDS) is an autosomal dominant syndrome characterized by the presence of firm skin-colored papules on the face, neck, and chest, and the development of lung cysts, pneumothorax, and renal cell carcinoma.[1–7] The syndrome was initially described in 1977,[8] and has been sometimes referred to as Hornstein-Knickenberg syndrome.[9] Biopsy of a firm facial papule reveals a diagnosis of fibrofol-liculoma or trichodiscoma,[8,10] which should raise the consideration for the diagnosis. In addition to the flesh-colored papules, patients can also have soft pedunculated skin taglike growths on the neck.[1,7] Patients with BHDS have numerous pulmonary diseases, including pneumothorax, lung cysts, and bullous emphysema.[5,11,12] Renal tumors are definitively associated with BHDS, but anecdotal reports have also linked other malignancies.

Clinical presentation

The typical patient with BHDS will develop skin-colored papules on the face (**Figs. 1** and **2**), neck, and chest after the age of 30 years. The papules are small (2–4 mm),

---

Department of Dermatology, Columbia University, 161 Fort Washington Avenue, Herbert Irving Pavilion, 12th Floor, New York, NY 10032, USA
* Corresponding author.
E-mail address: ru2111@columbia.edu (R. Ubriani).

Med Clin N Am 93 (2009) 1305–1331
doi:10.1016/j.mcna.2009.08.002
0025-7125/09/$ – see front matter © 2009 Elsevier Inc. All rights reserved.

Table 1
Color and texture of facial papules with underlying disorder and associated malignancies

Clinical Description	Underlying Disorder	Associated Malignancies
Flesh-colored	Birt-Hogg-Dubé syndrome	Renal
	Basal cell nevus syndrome	Medulloblastoma, craniopharyngioma, meningioma, fetal rhabdomyoma
	Neurofibromatosis, type 1	Gliomas, soft tissue sarcomas, myelogenous leukemia, breast cancer, generally increased risk of malignancy
Warty	Cowden syndrome	Breast, thyroid, endometrial, cerebellar
Waxy	Amyloid	Monoclonal gammopathy of undetermined significance, multiple myeloma
Red-yellow	Tuberous sclerosis	Hamartomas, astrocytomas, glioblastomas, cardiac rhabdomyomas, renal angiomyolipomas, renal cell carcinoma, pulmonary lymphangioleiomyomatosis
Red-yellow	Multiple endocrine neoplasia, type I	Pituitary (multiple), parathyroid adenomas, enteropancreatic (multiple), carcinoid, leiomyomas
Red-brown	Multicentric reticulohistiocytosis	Varied
Yellow	Muir-Torre syndrome	Colorectal, genitourinary, breast, lung, hematologic, others reported
Yellow	Necrobiotic xanthogranuloma	Monoclonal paraproteinemia, multiple myeloma, plasma cell dyscrasia, lymphoproliferative disorder

smooth, dome-shaped, flesh-colored to yellowish white, and usually asymptomatic. They affect the face, neck, chest, and oral cavity,[13] and are numerous. Acrochordon, or skin tags, originally described as part of the syndrome, are a nonspecific cutaneous finding, or represent fibrofolliculomas.[14] All of the lesions in BHDS were initially described as white papules in white patients, but as the disease has since been observed in other ethnic groups, it is more accurate to describe them as flesh-colored.[15]

Etiology

BHDS is an autosomal dominant inherited disease mapped to the short arm of chromosome 17 (17p11.2). Germline mutations in the BHD gene, also known as FLCN, are the cause of the disease. The gene contains 14 exons.[16] Most of the identified mutations lead to frameshift or nonsense mutations that cause truncation of the protein folliculin.[15–17] A folliculin-interacting protein has been identified and named FNIP1.[18] It has been found to interact with 5′-AMP–activated protein kinase, which negatively regulates the mammalian target of rapamycin, a high-level regulator for cell growth and proliferation.[18] This may be the mechanism for increased cancer in BHDS.

Pathologic findings

The distinctive pathologic finding is fibrofolliculoma, a tumor of the hair follicle that appears as cords and strands emanating from a central follicle.[10] Trichodiscomas and other pathologic findings have been described with BHDS, but it seems that these are more likely fibrofolliculomas that have been sectioned in a way that obscures the true pathologic finding.[7,14]

Associated malignancy

Patients with BHDS are 7 times more likely to develop renal cell carcinoma, according to a large case-control study.[12] Patients with BHDS develop renal tumors that are more frequently multiple and bilateral.[12,19] Chromophobe renal carcinoma, an otherwise rare kidney cancer, was the most common renal tumor in that same study. The largest analysis of renal tumors to date showed that renal tumors were chromophobe renal cell carcinomas (34%), hybrid oncocytic neoplasms (50%), or conventional clear cell renal carcinomas (9%).[20] Anecdotal reports have linked BHDS with medullary thyroid carcinoma,[8] neural tissue tumors,[21] connective tissue nevus,[22] intestinal polyposis,[23,24] lipomas, angiolipomas, parathyroid adenomas,[25] and parotid oncocytoma.[26] The largest case-control series showed no statistically significant evidence of increased medullary thyroid carcinoma, colon cancer, or intestinal polyposis.[12]

Basal Cell Nevus Syndrome

Overview

Basal cell nevus syndrome (BCNS), also known as nevoid basal cell carcinoma syndrome, Gorlin syndrome, or Gorlin-Goltz syndrome, was first described in 1960.[27] It is an autosomal dominant disorder characterized by the presence of multiple basal cell carcinomas (BCC) mostly in sun-exposed locations, a characteristic facies, jaw cysts, pits on the palms and soles, skeletal abnormalities, and the development of medulloblastoma.[28–30]

Clinical presentation

The typical patient with BCNS develops multiple flesh-colored to pigmented papules on the central face (**Figs. 3** and **4**) in the mid-20s. Lesions tend to be numerous and stable until puberty when they can enlarge and become more aggressive.[31] Although African American patients can develop the disorder, they develop the basal cell cancers at a much lower rate and these will not usually be detected from examination of facial papules.[31,32] Patients tend to have a distinctive coarse facies, with macrocephaly, frontal bossing, and hypertelomerism. Cleft lip or cleft palate has been noted in about 5% of cases.[28,31] Patients tend to develop multiple large epidermal cysts on the extremities. Small pits on the palms and soles are present in most cases. Soaking the hands in water for about 10 minutes makes the pits more obvious.[28,31,33] Patients develop multiple odontogenic keratocysts of the jaw that tend to occur early in life, more often in the mandible than the maxilla.[28] Skeletal and radiologic findings include lamellar calcification of the falx cerebri and splayed or bifid ribs.[28,31]

Etiology

BCNS is an autosomal dominant inherited disease mapped to chromosome 9q22.3.[34] Mutations in the gene Patched are the cause of the disease. New mutations account for about 50% of the cases.[28] Mutations in Patched prevent the attachment of Sonic Hedgehog. In the absence of this attachment, Patched cannot perform its usual role of inhibiting the protein Smoothened. Left uninhibited, Smoothened is freed for downstream signaling and growth promotion. In effect, mutations in Patched cause problems in tumor suppression.[28,35]

Table 2
Disorders discussed with clinical characteristics, cause, and associated malignancy

Diagnosis	Age at Presentation	Clinical Appearance of Lesions	Distribution of Lesions	Histopathology of Facial papules	Cause	Associated Malignancy
Birt-Hogg-Dubé syndrome	25–30 y	2–4 mm smooth white dome-shaped papules ± acrochordonlike lesions	Face, neck, chest, oral cavity	Fibrofolliculoma, trichodiscoma	Genetic, autosomal dominant, 17p11.2, BHD or FLCN gene encoding folliculin	Renal cell carcinoma (chromophobe, hybrid oncocytic, clear cell)
Basal cell nevus syndrome	10–20 y	Few to thousands of pearly white, flesh-colored, or pigmented papules	Sun-exposed face, neck, and chest	Basal cell carcinoma	Genetic, autosomal dominant, 9q22.3, PTCH gene encoding patched	Basal cell carcinoma, cardiac fibromas, fetal rhabdomyomas, desmoplastic medulloblastoma, craniophary-ngiomas, meningiomas, ovarian fibromas
Neurofibromatosis type 1	Childhood	Flesh-colored papules	Generalized	Neurofibroma	Genetic, autosomal dominant, 17q11.2, NF-1 gene encoding neurofibromin, a negative regulator of the Ras oncogene	Gliomas, soft tissue sarcomas, myelogenous leukemia, breast cancer, generally increased risk of malignancy
Cowden syndrome	Early to mid 20s	Warty papules	Face, localized near orifices	Trichilemmoma or nondistinctive	Genetic, autosomal dominant, 10q23.3, PTEN gene encoding a lipid phosphatase	Breast cancer, thyroid cancer (follicular or papillary), endometrial carcinoma, dysplastic gangliocytoma of the cerebellum (Lhermitte-Duclos disease)

Amyloid	Elderly, male 2:1	Waxy coalescing papules, sometimes associated with hemorrhage	Face, located near orifices	Amorphous pink eosinophilic fissured material	Immunologic, plasma cell dyscrasia producing light chain proteins that misfold into aggregates of amyloid protein	Monoclonal gammopathy of undetermined significance, multiple myeloma
Tuberous sclerosis	Childhood, first decade of life	Red-yellow discrete papules	Symmetrically located on the side of the nose, forehead, cheeks, and chin	Increased fibrous tissue oriented perpendicularly and around dilated blood vessels	Genetic, autosomal dominant, 9q34, TSC1, encoding hamartin, or 16p13, TSC2, encoding tuberin, a negative regulator of Rap1 and Rab5, which slow endocytosis	Various hamartomas, especially in the brain and retina, giant cell astrocytomas, glioblastomas, cardiac rhabdomyomas, renal angiomyolipomas, renal cell carcinoma, pulmonary lymphangioleiomyomatosis
Multiple endocrine neoplasia, type I	Not described	Red-yellow discrete papules	Upper lip	Increased fibrous tissue oriented perpendicularly and around dilated blood vessels	Genetic, autosomal dominant, 11q13, MEN1, encoding menin, a tumor suppressor	Pituitary tumors, parathyroid adenomas, enteropancreatic tumors, carcinoid tumors, leiomyomas

(continued on next page)

Table 2
(continued)

Diagnosis	Age at Presentation	Clinical Appearance of Lesions	Distribution of Lesions	Histopathology of Facial papules	Cause	Associated Malignancy
Multicentric reticulohistio-cytosis	40–50 y	1–20 mm red-brown papules and nodules	Ears, nose, nasal or oral mucosa, neck, trunk, hands, periungual	Dermal nodule made up of characteristic histiocytes and bizarre multinucleated giant cells	Believed to be inflammatory response to immune stimulus	Varied, about 25% will have underlying malignancy
Muir-Torre syndrome	40–50 y	Yellow papules of various sizes, dome-shaped papules with crateriform centers	Face, especially periorbital, neck, and chest	Spectrum of sebaceous growths including hyperplasia, adenoma, epithelioma, and carcinoma, which appear as sebaceous and basaloid proliferations with varying degrees of atypia	Genetic, autosomal dominant, 2p22-p21, encoding MSH2, 3p21.3, encoding MLH1, or 2p16, encoding MSH6. All proteins involved in DNA mismatch repair	Colorectal, genitourinary predominant, numerous other cancers, including breast, lung, and hematologic
Necrobiotic xantho-granuloma	50–60 y	Subcutaneous nodules or yellow plaques that can develop central atrophy	Face, especially periorbital, neck, trunk, proximal extremities	Palisading xanthogranuloma with zones of necrobiosis, giant cells, cholesterol clefts, lipid vacuoles	Unknown mechanism	Monoclonal paraproteinemia, multiple myeloma, plasma cell dyscrasia, lymphoproliferative disorder

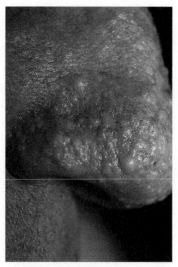

Fig. 1. Flesh-colored papules on the nose (BHDS).

Pathologic findings

Biopsy of a facial papule will demonstrate a BCC. The pathology is indistinguishable from BCC that develops in nonsyndromic patients. Nodular and superficial BCCs are the most common subtypes that will develop.[28]

Associated malignancy

BCCs number from a few to thousands on the face, neck, and chest. Although these have an extremely low rate of metastasis, they can cause significant morbidity due to local invasion and the need for repeated surgical procedures. Medulloblastomas tend to develop earlier than in the general population, are more often of the desmoplastic

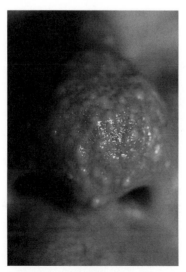

Fig. 2. Flesh-colored papules on the nose (BHDS).

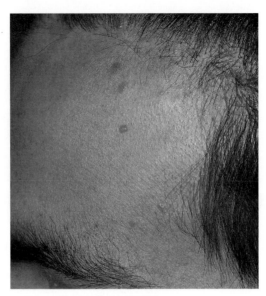

Fig. 3. Pigmented papules on the forehead (BCNS).

subtype, and occur at greater frequency in male patients with BCNS than in the general population.[36] Other brain tumors may develop, including meningioma and craniopharyngiomas (but this may be a consequence of radiation therapy for the diagnosis of medulloblastoma).[36] Three to 5% of BCNS patients develop cardiac fibromas. Although this is a benign tumor, it can cause arrhythmias.[37] Fetal rhabdomyoma may also develop. This tumor is extremely rare, comprising less than 2% of all neoplasms, showing striated muscle differentiation and is found predominantly in the head and neck region. It is a benign tumor that tends to present as a slow-growing mass, and

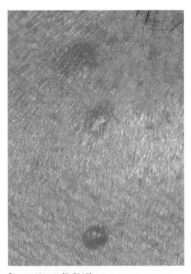

Fig. 4. Close-up of papules from **Fig. 3** (BCNS).

surgical excision is usually recommended.[38] Ovarian fibromas are present in about 20% of women affected by BCNS. They are more likely to be bilateral, large, calcified, and present at a younger age, with a mean age of 30 years at presentation in one study.[31,39] There are rare reports of development of ovarian fibrosarcoma,[40] ovarian leiomyosarcoma,[41] or virilizing stromal tumors.[42] Patients with BCNS do develop lymphatic and chylous mesenteric cysts, but the prevalence is not established. Odontogenic keratocysts are a major feature of the disease, developing in approximately two-thirds of patients, and they are frequently multiple and affect the upper and lower jaw. They are usually painless and present with swelling in most cases. These cysts can rarely develop ameloblastoma[43–46] or squamous cell carcinoma.[47] There are several other malignancies that have been associated with BCNS, but these have been isolated anecdotal reports and their significance is not known.[28]

Neurofibromatosis Type 1

Overview
Neurofibromatosis type 1 (NF-1), also known as von Recklinghausen disease, is an autosomal dominant disorder with numerous skin manifestations in addition to manifestations in the nervous system and bone. Patients are at increased risk for the development of numerous malignancies, especially malignant myeloid disorders.[48–52]

Clinical presentation
The diagnosis will usually be known by the time numerous facial papules develop, but subtle cases are sometimes noted late in life. The typical lesion is a soft, rubbery, flesh-colored papule or nodule (**Fig. 5**) that can be depressed into the underlying fat as through a buttonhole. It will spring back when pressure is removed. It is not unusual for unaffected patients to develop 1 neurofibroma, but the development of 2 or more should raise the possibility of neurofibromatosis and trigger a screening evaluation.[48] Most patients will have developed the cutaneous signs of neurofibromatosis by the second decade of life.[48,49,52]

Every organ system can be affected by neurofibromatosis, but physical signs for diagnostic criteria are: (1) 6 or more café-au-lait macules, greater than 5 mm in diameter before puberty or greater than 15 mm after puberty; (2) 2 or more neurofibromas or 1 plexiform neurofibroma; (3) freckling in the axillary or inguinal region (Crowe sign); (4) optic glioma; (5) 2 or more iris hamartomas (Lisch nodules); (6) a distinctive osseus lesion, such as dysplasia of the sphenoid bone behind the globe of the eye[53] (which

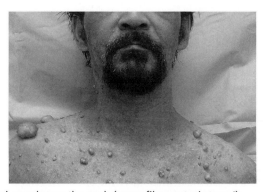

Fig. 5. Flesh-colored papules on the neck (neurofibromatosis type I).

can lead to exophthalmos) or thinning of the cortex of long bones with or without pseudarthrosis (non-natural articulation of the bone due to fracture and displacement).[54] An affected first-degree relative is another criterion. Diagnosis of NF-1 requires the presence of 2 or more of these criteria.[48]

Etiology

NF-1 is an autosomal dominant disorder mapped to chromosome 17q11.2.[55,56] Mutations in the gene NF1 are the cause of the disease and lead to dysfunctional neurofibromin protein.[55,56] New mutations account for about 50% of cases. Neurofibromin seems to function as a tumor suppressor, with the capacity to regulate multiple pathways including the Ras oncogene.[55,56] Inactivation of neurofibromin leads to increased activity of Ras and downstream signaling for increased cell growth.

Pathologic findings

Biopsy of the typical papule will demonstrate the diagnosis of neurofibroma. Well-circumscribed spindle cell proliferation with a mucinous background and mast cells are present.

Associated malignancy

Patients with NF-1 are at a 4 times increased risk for malignancy compared with the general population.[50,57,58] Patients are at significant risk for development of optic gliomas and other gliomas of the central nervous system. Neurofibromas can rarely develop into neurofibrosarcomas, and plexiform neurofibromas can develop malignant peripheral nerve sheath tumors. For this reason, any rapidly growing, hardening, or painful lesion in a patient with NF-1 warrants a biopsy.[59] NF-1 patients also have an increased rate of rhabdomyosarcoma.[60] The risk of myelogenous leukemia, especially juvenile chronic myelogenous leukemia, is elevated, even more so in the subset of patients with NF-1 and coexisting juvenile xanthogranulomas.[61] The reason for this association has not been determined, although it has been postulated that loss of p53 in addition to the NF-1 mutation may be the cause.[62] An increased risk of breast cancer has recently been reported; analysis showed that women younger than 50 years with NF-1 were 5 times as likely to develop breast cancer as unaffected women.[63] Associations with pheochromocytoma and gastrointestinal stromal tumors have also been reported.[64]

VERRUCOUS PAPULES
Cowden Syndrome

Overview

Cowden syndrome (CS), also known as multiple hamartoma syndrome, is an autosomal dominant syndrome, first described in 1962, characterized by the presence of multiple facial trichilemmomas, papillomas of the oral mucosa, and acral keratotic papules, and associated with the development of breast, endometrial, and thyroid carcinoma. The causative gene PTEN is also the causative gene for Bannayan-Riley-Ruvalcaba syndrome, Proteus syndrome, and Proteus-like syndrome, which share some clinical features with CS.[65–69]

Clinical presentation

Patients with CS typically present with skin findings in the second or third decade of life. Small, rough, warty papules in the central face and localized around orifices are the hallmark of the disease.[70] These lesions can also be smooth or dome-shaped. Most patients develop oral papillomas, which give the lips, tongue and gingiva a "cobblestone" appearance. Acral and palmoplantar keratoses also occur.[71] The disease has wide variability and new criteria for diagnosis may lead to changes in the frequency of skin findings as patients are diagnosed by other criteria in the future.

Etiology

CS is an autosomal dominant disorder usually caused by a mutation in PTEN, mapped to chromosome 10q23.3.[72] Eighty percent of CS cases are reportedly caused by mutations in PTEN.[73] Smaller, more recent, studies have found mutations in PTEN in a smaller percentage of patients with CS.[71] Analysis is complicated by the variability of the disease expression. PTEN mutations are also the cause in 60% of patients with Bannayan-Riley-Ruvalcaba syndrome, 20% of patient with Proteus syndrome, and 50% of patients with Proteus-like syndrome.[68] Although these disorders share some features, there are differing noted rates of malignancy, suggesting that further work will elucidate a more detailed understanding. Some have argued that all these disorders, or at least CS and Bannayan-Riley-Ruvalcaba syndrome, are simply 1 condition presenting variably at different ages, and that both conditions should be renamed PTEN hamartoma tumor syndrome.[65,67,68] PTEN encodes a lipid phosphatase that negatively regulates a cellular pathway that leads to increased cellular growth and survival. Loss of PTEN activates this pathway.

Pathologic findings

Most of the warty papules will be diagnosed as trichilemmomas. A significant minority of facial papules will have a nonspecific verrucous pattern, or be consistent with trichilemmoma but not diagnostic. The pathologic findings are hyperkeratosis with a downward lobular growth of clear cells with a thin rim of palisading basal cells.[74–76]

Associated malignancy

Patients with CS are significantly more likely to develop breast carcinoma, thyroid carcinoma, and endometrial carcinoma. The lifetime risk of breast cancer developing in women with CS is estimated to be about 25% to 50%.[77] As in the general population, ductal carcinomas are the most commonly observed malignant lesion in CS. In case series that looked at breast cancer risk, cases of bilateral breast cancer were reported.[77] Breast cancer has also been reported in male patients with CS.[78] The risk is high enough that some have argued for prophylactic bilateral mastectomy.[79] Benign breast disease such as fibroadenomas, apocrine metaplasia, microcysts, adenosis, and mammary hamartomalike lesions is usually extensive, bilateral, and present at an early age in CS.[80] Patients with CS have an estimated 3% to 10% risk of developing thyroid carcinoma, usually of the follicular or papillary subtype. Childhood onset of thyroid cancer has been reported. Endometrial cancer risk in CS patients is estimated at 5% to 10%, or 2 to 4 times higher than the general population.[70] This risk has not been clearly established.

Dysplastic gangliocytoma of the cerebellum, also known as Lhermitte-Duclos disease, is a rare slow-growing hamartoma of the cerebellum that presents with symptoms of increased intracranial pressure such as headache, nausea, vomiting, ataxia, or seizures.[81,82] Death can result from mass effect via obstructive hydrocephalus and subsequent herniation. The adult-onset form of this disease is intimately tied to a diagnosis of CS. A diagnosis of adult-onset Lhermitte-Duclos is highly suggestive of concurrent CS. Recent analysis reveals PTEN mutations in most patients with adult-onset Lhermitte-Duclos disease.[81]

There are several other malignancies that have been reported in association with CS, but their incidence is unknown. They include renal cell cancer, melanoma, colon cancer, bladder cancer, ovarian cancer, and cervical cancer. Evidence is insufficient at this time to determine whether any of these are definitively linked to a diagnosis of CS.[71]

WAXY PAPULES
Primary Systemic Amyloidosis

Overview
Amyloid is a protein deposited in the skin and other organs in several disease states. Soluble proteins aggregate as insoluble amyloid fibrils causing end-organ damage.[83] The soluble proteins that serve as the precursor for the misfolded amyloid protein can be normal or secondary to a disease process.[84] Relevant to the current topic is the diagnosis of light chain amyloid, in which a plasma cell dyscrasia produces vast quantities of immunoglobulin light chains that misfold into an amyloid protein called AL, which deposits in the skin, producing smooth shiny waxy papules, nodules, and plaques. This disease has overlap with monoclonal gammopathy of undetermined significance and multiple myeloma.[85]

Clinical presentation
Forty percent of patients with primary systemic amyloidosis develop cutaneous manifestations.[86] The average age of presentation in one large study was in the mid-60s.[84] Smooth shiny waxy papules appear in periorificial areas (**Fig. 6**). The translucent waxiness of the papules may be confused with tense vesicles on cursory examination. With continued appearance of lesions, papules coalesce to form larger plaques. Purpura and ecchymoses may accompany the waxy papules or appear spontaneously. These are a result of amyloid deposition in blood vessel walls leading to fragility. They can appear after minor trauma (stroking or pinching the skin), Valsalva maneuvers (coughing, vomiting, straining), or maneuvers that dependently position the head (as in a rectal biopsy). An enlarged tongue (macroglossia) with indentations from the teeth, sclerodermalike cutaneous infiltration, and alopecia may also appear.[86]

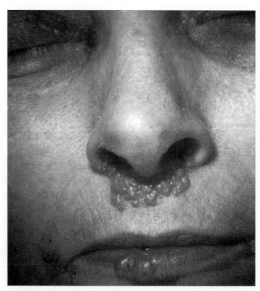

Fig. 6. Waxy papules on lower lip and nares, and purpuric papules on the eyelids (primary systemic amyloidosis associated with multiple myeloma).

Etiology

The source of the increased light chain protein that becomes the AL protein is usually a plasma cell dyscrasia related to multiple myeloma. Clonal plasma cells in the blood and bone marrow produce monoclonal light chains that have a tendency to misfold into a β-pleated sheet conformation of sheets of protein folded in an antiparallel fashion at alternating ends.[83–85] Lambda protein predominates, in a ratio that is the reverse of the normal state.[83] Certain light chain subtypes and amino acid substitutions have been found to predominate in amyloid protein, suggesting that these proteins may have a higher tendency to misfold because of molecular effects.[87] As this protein deposits in the skin, it produces the skin lesions described above. Deposition in vessels leads to fragility. Deposition is irregular and can affect all organs, leading to variable presentation that can include neuropathy, cardiomyopathy, nephrotic syndrome, adrenal insufficiency, hypothyroidism, dyspnea, bleeding, hepatomegaly, and other secondary effects from amyloid deposition.[83,84,86]

Pathologic findings

Biopsy of the facial papules will reveal pink eosinophilic fissured material that can be localized around blood vessels. Extravasated red blood cells may also be present. Special stains specific for amyloid, including Congo-red, thioflavin T, pagoda red, scarlet red, and periodic acid–Schiff, can be used to confirm the presence of amyloid. Congo-red staining will produce an orange-red stain under normal light and an apple-green birefringence under polarized light.[83,84]

Associated malignancy

The diagnosis of primary systemic amyloidosis with AL protein indicates an underlying plasma cell dyscrasia, which can include multiple myeloma or monoclonal gammopathy of undetermined significance. About 10% to 15% of patients with multiple myeloma will develop systemic amyloidosis, and a significant proportion of patients with systemic amyloidosis will have underlying multiple myeloma, but it is rare for patients with primary systemic amyloidosis and no evidence of multiple myeloma to progress to multiple myeloma at a later date.[88] Differing κ to λ ratios in primary systemic amyloidosis and multiple myeloma cases suggests distinct disorders.[84] Functional gene expression studies have also had success differentiating systemic amyloidosis from multiple myeloma.[89]

RED PAPULES
Tuberous Sclerosis

Overview

Tuberous sclerosis (TS), also known as Bourneville Disease,[90] is an autosomal dominant disorder with various manifestations in the skin, eyes, brain, bones, lungs, and kidneys. Patients have a high risk of hamartomas developing in the retina, brain, and kidney, but hamartomatous tumors can develop in nearly every organ of the body. A hamartoma is an overgrowth of normal cellular elements that is distinguished from a neoplasm by its lack of invasion or spread through the normal tissue. It tends to grow with the normal tissue.[91] Hamartomas can still cause significant disfigurement or pathophysiology by their mass effect.

Clinical presentation

The typical patient with TS will develop multiple red-yellow discrete facial papules (adenoma sebaceum) symmetrically on the sides of the nose, forehead, cheeks, and chin in the first decade of life.[92] A variant of angiofibroma, the fibrous plaque of the forehead, can be seen.[92] Nearly all patients will have hypopigmented ash-leaf shaped macules of the skin present at birth. Some patients will develop confettilike hypopigmented macules on the extremities.[93] About 50% of patients will develop a thickened patch of skin, a collagenoma (shagreen patch), most commonly on the lower back.[92,93] Oral examination may reveal small papules of the gingiva (cobblestoning) and multiple pits in the dental enamel.[94] About 50% of patients will have decreased intelligence of varying severity.[95] Nearly 80% will have seizures.[96]

Etiology

TS is an autosomal dominant inherited disease mapped to chromosomes 9q34 and 16p13. More than 50% of cases are due to spontaneous mutation. Mutations in the genes TSC1 (9q34) and TSC2 (16p13), respectively, are the cause of the disease. TSC1 encodes for the protein hamartin, which docks with tuberin, the protein product of TSC2.[90] The function of hamartin is unknown, but, based on its association with tuberin and the indistinguishable disease states that result from mutations in either, it is likely that it has a similar role to tuberin. Tuberin is believed to be a GTPase that negatively regulates the proteins Rap1 and Rab5 to slow the rate of endocytosis. Loss of tuberin function results in an increased rate of endocytosis, which may speed cell cycling.[91]

Pathologic findings

The red-yellow facial papules are angiofibromas on histopathology, making the classic term adenoma sebaceum a misnomer. A dome-shaped papule is seen with scattered dilated blood vessels in a network of increased collagen fibers, oriented around blood vessels and more perpendicularly in the upper layer of the skin.[97]

Associated malignancy

Most tumors in patients with TS are hamartomatous growths, but carcinomas can also develop. Patients with TS frequently develop retinal hamartomas[93] and, rarely, retinal astrocytomas.[98] Most patients will develop brain hamartomas that appear as multiple calcified nodules near the ventricles.[99] Similar lesions that continue to enlarge may be giant cell astrocytomas. When these are irradiated, patients can even develop glioblastomas.[100] Most patients will develop cardiac rhabdomyomas that can cause arrhythmias. These tend to involute spontaneously.[98] TS patients will almost always develop multiple bilateral renal angiomyolipomas, which can become symptomatic if they become large enough.[93] Renal cell carcinoma has also been reported in patients with TS.[101] Pulmonary lymphangioleiomyomatosis, a diffuse proliferation of smooth muscle cells in the lungs that can cause progressive dyspnea and pneumothorax, can occur as an infrequent complication of TS. It occurs almost exclusively in women of childbearing age.[102]

Multiple Endocrine Neoplasia, Type I

Overview

Multiple endocrine neoplasia type I (MEN-I), is a rare autosomal dominant disease first described by Wermer in 1954,[103] with skin findings similar to those of TS, and combinations of more than 20 different endocrine and nonendocrine tumors.[104,105]

Clinical presentation

Although facial angiofibromas were originally believed to be pathognomonic for TS, they have been reported to be present in MEN-I.[106] In a series of 32 patients, almost 90% had facial angiofibromas, and 50% had 5 or more.[106] The facial angiofibromas of MEN-I occur more frequently on the upper lip, an area that is less affected in TS.[106]

The age of presentation for these facial angiofibromas has not been described. Collagenomas (70%), café-au-lait macules, lipomas (30%), leiomyomas (10%), confettilike hypopigmented macules, and multiple gingival papules have also been described in patients with MEN-I.[107]

Etiology
MEN-I is an autosomal dominant inherited disease mapped to chromosome 11q13. Mutations in the MEN1 gene, which encodes the protein menin, are the cause of the disease. Menin seems to function as a tumor suppressor through the JunD transcription factor.[108]

Pathologic findings
The histopathology of the angiofibromas in MEN-I is indistinguishable from those found in TS.[106,109] These skin lesions demonstrate allelic deletion of the MEN1 gene.[110]

Associated malignancy
Patients with MEN-I develop pituitary, parathyroid, and pancreatic tumors, and carcinoid tumors, pheochromocytomas (rarely), and leiomyomas.[104,105] The most common pituitary tumors are prolactinomas, but growth hormone secreting tumors, adrenocorticotropic hormone secreting tumors, and nonfunctioning tumors can also develop.[105] Nearly all patients (90%) will develop primary hyperparathyroidism, most frequently multinodular hyperplasia. The age of onset for MEN-1–associated parathyroid adenoma is about 25 years, in contrast to sporadic cases of onset in the fifth decade.[104] Enteropancreatic tumors are various and present in about 60% of patients. The most common tumor is gastrinoma, which can be multiple and metastatic.[105] About half of MEN-I patients will develop gastrinomas by the age of 50 years.[105] Insulinomas, glucagonomas, vasoactive intestinal peptide-secreting tumors (VIPomas), somatostatinomas, and nonfunctioning tumors also occur.[105]

Most sporadic carcinoid tumors occur in the hindgut. In contrast, carcinoid tumors that develop in MEN-I develop in the foregut, and can also occur in unusual locations such as thymus, bronchus, and duodenum.[104,105] Pheochromocytoma is rare in MEN-I, but has been reported; it is more traditionally associated with multiple endocrine neoplasia, type II.[105]

Multicentric Reticulohistiocytosis

Overview
Multicentric reticulohistiocytosis (MRH) is an idiopathic inflammatory reaction that manifests as red-brown papules and a destructive polyarthritis. MRH is associated with a malignancy about 25% of the time.[111]

Clinical presentation
The typical patient with MRH is a middle-aged woman. Women develop MRH 2 to 3 times more often than men. Most cases have been reported in whites, but the disease seems to affect all races.[112] The cutaneous signs may precede or follow the arthritis, but are present in nearly all cases.[112] Reddish brown papules of a wide range of sizes appear on the face (with a predilection for the ears and nose), hands, neck, and trunk. Severe facial involvement can produce a leonine facies.[113] About 50% of patients will develop mucosal involvement, with papules on the lips, cheeks, tongue, gingival, or nasal septum.[113] On the hands, the papulonodules appear over the joints or on the proximal nail fold (periungual "coral bead" appearance).[114] The papules are usually

asymptomatic, but erythema and pruritus may precede their appearance in some cases.

Etiology
The disease is believed to be an inflammatory response to varied stimuli. Cases have been reported with systemic tuberculosis, malignancy, autoimmune disease, or with no clear underlying pathology.[113–115]

Pathologic findings
Histopathology of the lesions shows a well-defined dermal nodule composed of characteristic histiocytes and bizarre multinucleated giant cells with ground-glass cytoplasm. There is a scattered polymorphous cell infiltrate of lymphocytes, eosinophils, neutrophils, and plasma cells.[112]

Associated malignancy
About a quarter of cases are associated with an underlying malignancy. MRH has been reported in association with a variety of cancers including carcinoma of the breast, stomach, colon, ovary, and cervix, and leukemia and lymphoma.[111] The improvement of malignancy-associated MRH coincident with chemotherapy and the reappearance of MRH before a malignancy recurrence has been reported.[116] Appearance of MRH can precede the development of a tumor by months or years, and relapse of MRH can be a marker for tumor recurrence.

YELLOW PAPULES
Muir-Torre Syndrome

Overview
Muir-Torre syndrome (MTS), first described in 1967, is an autosomal dominant disease with cutaneous sebaceous neoplasms and keratoacanthomas, associated with 1 or more low-grade visceral malignancies.[35] Colorectal cancer is the most commonly observed visceral malignancy in MTS, followed by genitourinary cancer.[117]

Clinical presentation
Patients usually present in the fifth or sixth decade of life, although the age range of cases in the literature is as low as the early 20s.[118] Most cases have been noted in white patients. Patients develop numerous sebaceous tumors on the face, often in the periocular area. These typically present as yellow papules (**Fig. 7**) or nodules of various sizes. Patients also develop either solitary or multiple keratoacanthomas, which appear as domed papules with a central keratin-filled crater. The sebaceous tumors in MTS can precede, occur concurrently, or follow the diagnosis of internal malignancy.[117]

Etiology
MTS is an autosomal dominant disease mapped to chromosomes 2p and 3p21.3. Mutations in the genes MSH2 (2p22-p21) and MLH1 (3p21.3) account for most cases, with MSH2 being the more common cause.[119] More recently, MSH6 (2p16) mutations have been described in cases of MTS negative for MSH2 or MLH1 mutations.[120] These proteins are all implicated in hereditary nonpolyposis colorectal cancer (HNPCC), also known as Lynch syndrome. MTS is likely a phenotypic variant of HNPCC. All of these proteins are enzymes involved in DNA mismatch repair.[120] Loss of their function leads to accumulation of errors and lengthening or shortening of repeated sequences of DNA in the genome, a phenomenon known as microsatellite instability.[121]

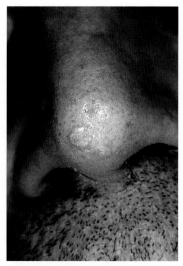

Fig. 7. Yellow papule on the nasal tip (Muir-Torre syndrome).

Pathologic findings

Yellow papules on the face are diagnosed as a spectrum of sebaceous growths including hyperplasia, adenoma, epithelioma, and carcinoma. Sebaceous adenomas, the most distinctive cutaneous marker for MTS, are a circumscribed lobular proliferation of mature sebaceous cells centrally, and basaloid cells peripherally, with little to no atypia. Sebaceous epithelioma and carcinoma are nearly as specific for MTS. Sebaceous epithelioma shows fewer sebaceous cells and increased basaloid cells. Sebaceous carcinoma is an aggressive-appearing, poorly defined proliferation of fewer sebaceous, and increased basaloid, cells with moderate to severe atypia and possible pagetoid spread.[117,122,123] A particular type of tumor called seboacanthoma is unique to MTS; it displays the dome-shaped nodule and central crater architecture of a keratoacanthoma, but is made up of sebaceous lobules.[35,117] Patients can also develop BCCs with sebaceous differentiation. There are sebaceous tumors of the skin that are not specific for MTS, such as sebaceous hyperplasia and nevus sebaceous of Jadassohn.[119]

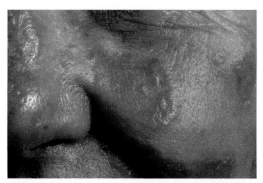

Fig. 8. Yellow irregular plaques with central atrophy on the cheek (necrobiotic xanthogranuloma).

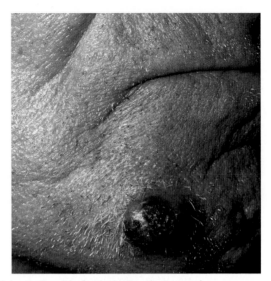

Fig. 9. Eroded nodule on the chin (metastatic colon cancer).

Associated malignancy

Patients with MTS develop a wide variety of malignancies, but most cancers are in the colorectal (50%) or genitourinary (25%) systems.[118] The colon cancer that develops in MTS tends to be proximal to the splenic flexure and develop a decade earlier than sporadic colon cancer. Numerous other cancers, including breast, lung, and hematologic, have been described. Multiple malignancies are common; in one large review, almost half of the patients had more than 1 visceral malignancy.[118] Despite affected patients having multiple malignancies, the sebaceous and visceral cancers of MTS are less aggressive than their non-MTS counterparts. As a result, MTS responds well to aggressive surgical management, affording a favorable prognosis with prolonged survival even in the presence of metastases.[119]

Necrobiotic Xanthogranuloma

Overview

Necrobiotic xanthogranuloma (NXG), first described in 1980, is a rare multisystem disease of unknown cause, which presents with eye and skin findings with a distinctive

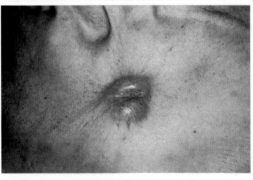

Fig. 10. Pink nodule on the cheek (metastatic breast cancer).

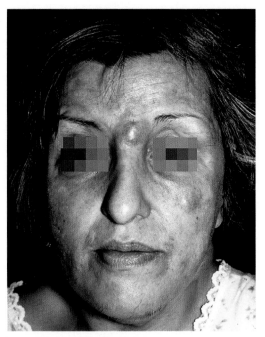

Fig. 11. Purple nodules on the face (lymphoma).

histopathologic appearance, and is associated with monoclonal paraproteinemias and hematologic malignancies.[124]

Clinical presentation
The typical patient with NXG is middle-aged. Men and women are affected equally. Yellowish or xanthomatous papules, nodules, and subcutaneous plaques develop on the face, neck, trunk, and proximal limbs. The periorbital region is the most common site of involvement. The plaques are yellow, irregular in shape, and can have central atrophy (**Fig. 8**) with scarring, telangiectasias, or ulceration.[124,125] The lesions are firm and indurated, and cause ophthalmologic manifestations in about 50% of cases. NXG can directly involve the orbit or cause inflammation of the eye.[126] Patients can develop mucosal involvement, lymphadenopathy, and hepatosplenomegaly. NXG may involve extracutaneous sites including the heart, lungs, kidney, larynx, pharynx, intestine, ovary, skeletal muscle, and the central nervous system.[124,125]

Etiology
The cause of NXG is unknown.

Pathologic findings
Biopsy specimens from a plaque show large areas of degenerated collagen surrounded by palisaded macrophages. The granulomatous process extends through the fat and contains foamy histiocytes, lymphocytes, plasma cells, and neutrophils. Prominent Touton giant cells, foreign body giant cells, and large and bizarre angulated giant cells are present, adjacent to areas of degenerated collagen, which may contain cholesterol clefts and lipid vacuoles.[112,122]

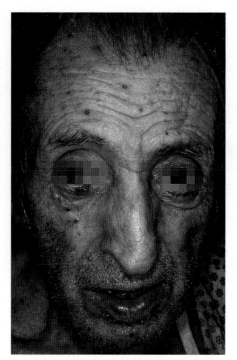

Fig. 12. Numerous black papules on the face (metastatic malignant melanoma).

Associated malignancy

Most cases (80%–90%) have an associated monoclonal paraproteinemia,[126,127] most frequently IgG κ (60%) and IgG λ (26%), and only rarely IgA.[128] Only a few patients develop multiple myeloma (approximately 10%).[129] Other lymphoproliferative disorders and malignancies may be present, including Hodgkin disease, non-Hodgkin lymphoma, chronic lymphocytic leukemia,[130] myelodysplastic syndrome, amyloidosis, macroglobulinemia, and cryoglobulinemia.[125]

Cutaneous metastases

Any unexplained facial papule(s) or nodule(s) may be a presenting sign of internal malignancy (**Fig. 9**).[131,132] Red papules or "vascular" papules may be renal or thyroid cancer metastases. Skin-colored, pink, or red papules may be breast or lung cancer metastases (**Fig. 10**). Skin-colored, pink, purple, or plum-colored papules may represent leukemic or lymphomatous infiltrates (**Fig. 11**). Black papules are metastatic malignant melanoma (**Fig. 12**).[131–134] In all cases, skin biopsy in conjunction with immunoperoxidase stains is usually diagnostic of the primary malignancy.[135,136]

REFERENCES

1. Adley BP, Smith ND, Nayar R, et al. Birt-Hogg-Dubé syndrome: clinicopathologic findings and genetic alterations. Arch Pathol Lab Med 2006;130:1865–70.
2. Gruson LM. Birt-Hogg-Dube syndrome. Dermatol Online J 2004;10:15.
3. Haimowitz JE, Halpern AC, Heymann WR. Multiple, hereditary dome-shaped papules and acrochordons. Birt-Hogg-Dubé syndrome. Arch Dermatol 1997; 133:1163–6.

4. Kupres KA, Krivda SJ, Turiansky GW. Numerous asymptomatic facial papules and multiple pulmonary cysts: a case of Birt-Hogg-Dubé syndrome. Cutis 2003;72(2):127–31.
5. Leter EM, Koopmans AK, Gille JJ, et al. Birt-Hogg-Dubé syndrome: clinical and genetic studies of 20 families. J Invest Dermatol 2008;128:45–9.
6. Schmidt LS, Warren MB, Nickerson ML, et al. Birt-Hogg-Dubé syndrome, a genodermatosis associated with spontaneous pneumothorax and kidney neoplasia, maps to chromosome 17p11.2. Am J Hum Genet 2001;69:876–82.
7. Vincent A, Farley M, Chan E, et al. Birt-Hogg-Dubé syndrome: a review of the literature and the differential diagnosis of firm facial papules. J Am Acad Dermatol 2003;49(4):698–705.
8. Birt AR, Hogg GR, Dubé WJ. Hereditary multiple fibrofolliculomas with trichodiscomas and acrochordons. Arch Dermatol 1977;113:1674–7.
9. Schulz T, Hartschuh W. Birt-Hogg-Dubé syndrome and Hornstein-Knickenberg syndrome are the same. Different sectioning technique as the cause of different histology. J Cutan Pathol 1999;26:55–61.
10. Collins GL, Somach S, Morgan MB. Histomorphologic and immunophenotypic analysis of fibrofolliculomas and trichodiscomas in Birt-Hogg-Dube syndrome and sporadic disease. J Cutan Pathol 2002;29:529–33.
11. Toro JR, Pautler SE, Stewart L, et al. Lung cysts, spontaneous pneumothorax, and genetic associations in 89 families with Birt-Hogg-Dubé syndrome. Am J Respir Crit Care Med 2007;175:1044–53.
12. Zbar B, Alvord WG, Glenn G, et al. Risk of renal and colonic neoplasms and spontaneous pneumothorax in the Birt-Hogg-Dubé syndrome. Cancer Epidemiol Biomarkers Prev 2002;11(4):393–400.
13. Nadershahi NA, Wescott WB, Egbert B. Birt-Hogg-Dubé syndrome: a review and presentation of the first case with oral lesions. Oral Surg Oral Med Oral Pathol Oral Radiol Endod 1997;83:496–500.
14. De la Torre C, Ocampo C, Doval IG, et al. Acrochordons are not a component of the Birt-Hogg-Dubé syndrome: does this syndrome exist? Case reports and review of the literature. Am J Dermatopathol 1999;21:369–74.
15. Kim EH, Jeong SY, Kim HJ, et al. A case of Birt-Hogg-Dubé syndrome. J Korean Med Sci 2008;23:332–5.
16. Khoo SK, Bradley M, Wong FK, et al. Birt-Hogg-Dubé syndrome: mapping of a novel hereditary neoplasia gene to chromosome 17p12-q11.2. Oncogene 2001;20:5239–42.
17. Van Slegtenhorst M, Khabibullin D, Hartman TR, et al. The Birt-Hogg-Dube and tuberous sclerosis complex homologs have opposing roles in amino acid homeostasis in schizosaccharomyces pombe. J Biol Chem 2007;282(34): 24583–90.
18. Baba M, Furihata M, Hong SB, et al. Kidney-targeted Birt-Hogg-Dube gene inactivation in a mouse model: Erk1/2 and Akt-mTOR activation, cell hyperproliferation, and polycystic kidneys. J Natl Cancer Inst 2008;100:140–54.
19. Roth JS, Rabinowitz AD, Benson M, et al. Bilateral renal cell carcinoma in the Birt-Hogg-Dubé syndrome. J Am Acad Dermatol 1993;29:1055–6.
20. Pavlovich CP, Walther MM, Eyler RA, et al. Renal tumors in the Birt-Hogg-Dubé syndrome. Am J Surg Pathol 2002;26:1542–52.
21. Vincent A, Farley M, Chan E, et al. Birt-Hogg-Dubé syndrome: two patients with neural tissue tumors. J Am Acad Dermatol 2003;49:717–9.
22. Weintraub R, Pinkus H. Multiple fibrofolliculomas (Birt-Hogg-Dubé) associated with a large connective tissue nevus. J Cutan Pathol 1977;4:289–99.

23. Rongioletti F, Hazini R, Gianotti G, et al. Fibrofolliculomas, tricodiscomas and acrochordons (Birt-Hogg-Dubé) associated with intestinal polyposis. Clin Exp Dermatol 1989;14:72–4.

24. Le Guyadec T, Dufau JP, Poulain JF, et al. [Multiple trichodiscomas associated with colonic polyposis]. Ann Dermatol Venereol 1998;125(10):717–9 [French].

25. Chung JY, Ramos-Caro FA, Beers B, et al. Multiple lipomas, angiolipomas, and parathyroid adenomas in a patient with Birt-Hogg-Dube syndrome. Int J Dermatol 1996;35:365–7.

26. Liu V, Kwan T, Page EH. Parotid oncocytoma in the Birt-Hogg-Dubé syndrome. J Am Acad Dermatol 2000;43:1120–2.

27. Gorlin RJ, Chaudhary AP. Multiple osteomatosis, fibromas, lipomas and fibrosarcomas of the skin and mesentery, epidermoid inclusion cysts of the skin, leiomyomas and multiple intestinal polyposis: a heritable disorder of connective tissue. N Engl J Med 1960;263:1151–8.

28. Gorlin RJ. Nevoid basal cell carcinoma (Gorlin) syndrome. Genet Med 2004;6:530–9.

29. Gorlin RJ. Nevoid basal-cell carcinoma syndrome. Medicine (Baltimore) 1987; 66:98–113.

30. Gorlin RJ, Sedano HO. The multiple nevoid basal cell carcinoma syndrome revisited. Birth Defects Orig Artic Ser 1971;7:140–8.

31. Kimonis VE, Goldstein AM, Pastakia B, et al. Clinical manifestations in 105 persons with nevoid basal cell carcinoma syndrome. Am J Med Genet 1997; 69:299–308.

32. Hall J, Johnston KA, McPhillips JP, et al. Nevoid basal cell carcinoma syndrome in a black child. J Am Acad Dermatol 1998;38:363–5.

33. Lo Muzio L. Nevoid basal cell carcinoma syndrome (Gorlin syndrome). Orph J Rare Dis 2008;3:32.

34. Farndon PA, Del Mastro RG, Evans DG, et al. Location of gene for Gorlin syndrome. Lancet 1992;339:581–2.

35. Burgdorf WH. Cancer-associated genodermatoses: a personal history. Exp Dermatol 2006;15:653–66.

36. Fukushima Y, Oka H, Utsuki S, et al. Nevoid basal cell carcinoma syndrome with medulloblastoma and meningioma–case report. Neurol Med Chir (Tokyo) 2004; 44:665–8.

37. Bossert T, Walther T, Vondrys D, et al. Cardiac fibroma as an inherited manifestation of nevoid basal-cell carcinoma syndrome. Tex Heart Inst J 2006;33: 88–90.

38. Watson J, Depasquale K, Ghaderi M, et al. Nevoid basal cell carcinoma syndrome and fetal rhabdomyoma: a case study. Ear Nose Throat J 2004;83:716–8.

39. Fonseca RB, Grzeszczak EF. Case 128: bilateral ovarian fibromas in nevoid basal cell carcinoma syndrome. Radiology 2008;246:318–21.

40. Kraemer BB, Silva EG, Sneige N. Fibrosarcoma of ovary. A new component in the nevoid basal-cell carcinoma syndrome. Am J Surg Pathol 1984;8: 231–6.

41. Seracchioli R, Colombo FM, Bagnoli A, et al. Primary ovarian leiomyosarcoma as a new component in the nevoid basal cell carcinoma syndrome: a case report. Am J Obstet Gynecol 2003;188:1093–5.

42. Ismail SM, Walker SM. Bilateral virilizing sclerosing stromal tumours of the ovary in a pregnant woman with Gorlin's syndrome: implications for pathogenesis of ovarian stromal neoplasms. Histopathology 1990;17:159–63.

43. Aithal D, Reddy BS, Mahajan S, et al. Ameloblastomatous calcifying odontogenic cyst: a rare histologic variant. J Oral Pathol Med 2003;32:376–8.

44. Dalati T, Zhou H. Gorlin syndrome with ameloblastoma: a case report and review of literature. Cancer Invest 2008;26:975–6.
45. Eslami B, Lorente C, Kieff D, et al. Ameloblastoma associated with the nevoid basal cell carcinoma (Gorlin) syndrome. Oral Surg Oral Med Oral Pathol Oral Radiol Endod 2008;105:e10–3.
46. Kamboj M, Juneja M. Ameloblastomatous Gorlin's cyst. J Oral Sci 2007;49: 319–23.
47. Ota Y, Karakida K, Watanabe D, et al. A case of central carcinoma of the mandible arising from a recurrent odontogenic keratocyst: delineation of surgical margins and reconstruction with bilateral rectus abdominis myocutaneous free flaps. Tokai J Exp Clin Med 1998;23:157–65.
48. Friedman JM. Neurofibromatosis 1: clinical manifestations and diagnostic criteria. J Child Neurol 2002;17:548–54.
49. Korf BR. Clinical features and pathobiology of neurofibromatosis 1. J Child Neurol 2002;17:573–7 [discussion: 602–74, 646–51].
50. Matsui I, Tanimura M, Kobayashi N, et al. Neurofibromatosis type 1 and childhood cancer. Cancer 1993;72:2746–54.
51. Upadhyaya M, Han S, Consoli C, et al. Characterization of the somatic mutational spectrum of the neurofibromatosis type 1 (NF1) gene in neurofibromatosis patients with benign and malignant tumors. Hum Mutat 2004; 23:134–46.
52. Young H, Hyman S, North K. Neurofibromatosis 1: clinical review and exceptions to the rules. J Child Neurol 2002;17:613–21 [discussion: 627–19, 646–51].
53. Caldemeyer K. Neurofibromatosis type 1. Part I. Clinical and central nervous system manifestations. J Am Acad Dermatol 2001;44:1025–6.
54. Bernauer TA, Mirowski GW, Caldemeyer KS. Neurofibromatosis type 1. Part II. Non-head and neck findings. J Am Acad Dermatol 2001;44:1027–9.
55. Gutmann DH, Wood DL, Collins FS. Identification of the neurofibromatosis type 1 gene product. Proc Natl Acad Sci U S A 1991;88:9658–62.
56. Marchuk DA, Saulino AM, Tavakkol R, et al. cDNA cloning of the type 1 neurofibromatosis gene: complete sequence of the NF1 gene product. Genomics 1991;11:931–40.
57. Korf B. Malignancy in neurofibromatosis type 1. Oncologist 2000;5:477–85.
58. Sørensen SA, Mulvihill JJ, Nielsen A. Long-term follow-up of von Recklinghausen neurofibromatosis. Survival and malignant neoplasms. N Engl J Med 1986;314: 1010–5.
59. Leroy K, Dumas V, Martin-Garcia N, et al. Malignant peripheral nerve sheath tumors associated with neurofibromatosis type 1: a clinicopathologic and molecular study of 17 patients. Arch Dermatol 2001;137:908–13.
60. Yang P, Grufferman S, Khoury MJ, et al. Association of childhood rhabdomyosarcoma with neurofibromatosis type I and birth defects. Genet Epidemiol 1995;12: 467–74.
61. Zvulunov A, Barak Y, Metzker A. Juvenile xanthogranuloma, neurofibromatosis, and juvenile chronic myelogenous leukemia. World statistical analysis. Arch Dermatol 1995;131:904–8.
62. Luria D, Avigad S, Cohen IJ, et al. p53 mutation as the second event in juvenile chronic myelogenous leukemia in a patient with neurofibromatosis type 1. Cancer 1997;80:2013–8.
63. Sharif S, Moran A, Huson SM, et al. Women with neurofibromatosis 1 are at a moderately increased risk of developing breast cancer and should be considered for early screening. J Med Genet 2007;44:481–4.

64. Zoeller MET, Rembeck B, Oden A, et al. Malignant and benign tumors in patients with neurofibromatosis type 1 in a defined Swedish population. Cancer 1997;79: 2125–31.

65. Yin Y, Shen WH. PTEN: a new guardian of the genome. Oncogene 2008;27: 5443–53.

66. Orloff MS, Eng C. Genetic and phenotypic heterogeneity in the PTEN hamartoma tumour syndrome. Oncogene 2008;27:5387–97.

67. Blumenthal GM, Dennis PA. PTEN hamartoma tumor syndromes. Eur J Hum Genet 2008;16:1289–300.

68. Eng C. PTEN: one gene, many syndromes. Hum Mutat 2003;22:183–98.

69. Marsh DJ, Kum JB, Lunetta KL, et al. PTEN mutation spectrum and genotype-phenotype correlations in Bannayan-Riley-Ruvalcaba syndrome suggest a single entity with Cowden syndrome. Hum Mol Genet 1999;8:1461–72.

70. Pilarski R, Eng C. Will the real Cowden syndrome please stand up (again)? Expanding mutational and clinical spectra of the PTEN hamartoma tumour syndrome. J Med Genet 2004;41:323–6.

71. Pilarski R. Cowden syndrome: a critical review of the clinical literature. J Genet Couns 2008;18:13–27.

72. Nelen MR, Padberg GW, Peeters EA, et al. Localization of the gene for Cowden disease to chromosome 10q22-23. Nat Genet 1996;13:114–6.

73. Marsh DJ, Coulon V, Lunetta KL, et al. Mutation spectrum and genotype-phenotype analyses in Cowden disease and Bannayan-Zonana syndrome, two hamartoma syndromes with germline PTEN mutation. Hum Mol Genet 1998;7:507–15.

74. Starink TM, Meijer CJ, Brownstein MH. The cutaneous pathology of Cowden's disease: new findings. J Cutan Pathol 1985;12:83–93.

75. Starink TM, Hausman R. The cutaneous pathology of facial lesions in Cowden's disease. J Cutan Pathol 1984;11:331–7.

76. Brownstein MH, Mehregan AH, Bikowski JB, et al. The dermatopathology of Cowden's syndrome. Br J Dermatol 1979;100:667–73.

77. Starink TM, van der Veen JP, Arwert F, et al. The Cowden syndrome: a clinical and genetic study in 21 patients. Clin Genet 1986;29:222–33.

78. Fackenthal JD, Marsh DJ, Richardson AL, et al. Male breast cancer in Cowden syndrome patients with germline PTEN mutations. J Med Genet 2001;38: 159–64.

79. Walton BJ, Morain WD, Baughman RD, et al. Cowden's disease: a further indication for prophylactic mastectomy. Surgery 1986;99:82–6.

80. Schrager CA, Schneider D, Gruener AC, et al. Clinical and pathological features of breast disease in Cowden's syndrome: an underrecognized syndrome with an increased risk of breast cancer. Hum Pathol 1998;29:47–53.

81. Abel TW, Baker SJ, Fraser MM, et al. Lhermitte-Duclos disease: a report of 31 cases with immunohistochemical analysis of the PTEN/AKT/mTOR pathway. J Neuropathol Exp Neurol 2005;64:341–9.

82. Prabhu SS, Aldape KD, Bruner JM, et al. Cowden disease with Lhermitte-Duclos disease: case report. Can J Neurol Sci 2004;31:542–9.

83. Falk RH, Comenzo RL, Skinner M. The systemic amyloidoses. N Engl J Med 1997;337:898–909.

84. Obici L, Perfetti V, Palladini G, et al. Clinical aspects of systemic amyloid diseases. Biochim Biophys Acta 2005;1753:11–22.

85. Hirschfield GM. Amyloidosis: a clinico-pathophysiological synopsis. Semin Cell Dev Biol 2004;15:39–44.

86. Breathnach SM. Amyloid and amyloidosis. J Am Acad Dermatol 1988;18:1–16.
87. Dhodapkar MV, Merlini G, Solomon A. Biology and therapy of immunoglobulin deposition diseases. Hematol Oncol Clin North Am 1997;11:89–110.
88. Rajkumar SV, Gertz MA, Kyle RA. Primary systemic amyloidosis with delayed progression to multiple myeloma. Cancer 1998;82:1501–5.
89. Abraham RS, Ballman KV, Dispenzieri A, et al. Functional gene expression analysis of clonal plasma cells identifies a unique molecular profile for light chain amyloidosis. Blood 2005;105:794–803.
90. Narayanan V. Tuberous sclerosis complex: genetics to pathogenesis. Pediatr Neurol 2003;29:404–9.
91. Kwiatkowski DJ. Tuberous sclerosis: from tubers to mTOR. Ann Hum Genet 2003; 67:87–96.
92. Webb DW, Carke A, Fyer A, et al. The cutaneous features of tuberous sclerosis: a population study. Br J Dermatol 1996;135:1–5.
93. Schwartz R, Fernandez G, Kotulska K, et al. Tuberous sclerosis complex: advances in diagnosis, genetics, and management. J Am Acad Dermatol 2007;57:189–202.
94. Sparling J, Hong C, Brahim J, et al. Oral findings in 58 adults with tuberous sclerosis complex. J Am Acad Dermatol 2007;56:786–90.
95. Jozwiak S, Goodman M, Lamm SH. Poor mental development in patients with tuberous sclerosis complex: clinical risk factors. Arch Neurol 1998;55:379–84.
96. Holmes GL, Stafstrom CE, Group TSS. Tuberous sclerosis complex and epilepsy: recent developments and future challenges. Epilepsia 2007;48:617–30.
97. Schaffer JV, Gohara MA, McNiff JM, et al. Multiple facial angiofibromas: a cutaneous manifestation of Birt-Hogg-Dubé syndrome. J Am Acad Dermatol 2005; 53:S108–11.
98. Bader RS, Chitayat D, Kelly E, et al. Fetal rhabdomyoma: prenatal diagnosis, clinical outcome, and incidence of associated tuberous sclerosis complex. J Pediatr 2003; 143:620–4.
99. Lin D, Barker P. Neuroimaging of phakomatoses. Semin Pediatr Neurol 2006;13: 48–62.
100. Matsumara H, Takimoto H, Shimada N, et al. Glioblastoma following radiotherapy in a patient with tuberous sclerosis: case report. Neurol Med Chir (Tokyo) 1998;38: 287–91.
101. Winship IM, Dudding TE. Lessons from the skin – cutaneous features of familial cancer. Lancet Oncol 2008;9:462–72.
102. Vicente M, Pons M, Medina M. Pulmonary involvement in tuberous sclerosis. Pediatr Pulmonol 2004;37:178–80.
103. Hoang-Xuan T, Steger JW. Adult-onset angiofibroma and multiple endocrine neoplasia type I. J Am Acad Dermatol 1999;41(5 Pt 2):890–2.
104. Zarnegar R, Brunaud L, Clark OH. Multiple endocrine neoplasia type I. Curr Treat Options Oncol 2002;3:335–48.
105. Schussheim DH, Skarulis MC, Agarwal SK, et al. Multiple endocrine neoplasia type 1: new clinical and basic findings. Trends Endocrinol Metab 2001;12: 173–8.
106. Darling TN, Skarulis MC, Steinberg SM, et al. Multiple facial angiofibromas and collagenomas in patients with multiple endocrine neoplasia type 1. Arch Dermatol 1997;133:853–7.
107. Vidal A, Iglesias M, Fernández B, et al. Cutaneous lesions associated to multiple endocrine neoplasia syndrome type 1. J Eur Acad Dermatol Venereol 2008;22: 835–8.

108. Marx S. Molecular genetics of multiple endocrine neoplasia types 1 and 2. Nat Rev Cancer 2005;5:367–75.

109. Asgharian B. Cutaneous tumors in patients with multiple endocrine neoplasm type 1 (MEN1) and gastrinomas: prospective study of frequency and development of criteria with high sensitivity and specificity for MEN1. J Clin Endocrinol Metab 2004;89:5328–36.

110. Pack S, Turner ML, Zhuang Z, et al. Cutaneous tumors in patients with multiple endocrine neoplasia type 1 show allelic deletion of the MEN1 gene. J Invest Dermatol 1998;110:438–40.

111. Nunnink JC, Krusinski PA, Yates JW. Multicentric reticulohistiocytosis and cancer: a case report and review of the literature. Med Pediatr Oncol 1985; 13:273–9.

112. Rapini RP. Multicentric reticulohistiocytosis. Clin Dermatol 1993;11:107–11.

113. Tajirian A, Malik M, Robinsonbostom L, et al. Multicentric reticulohistiocytosis. Clin Dermatol 2006;24:486–92.

114. Kalajian AH, Callen JP. Multicentric reticulohistiocytosis successfully treated with infliximab: an illustrative case and evaluation of cytokine expression supporting anti-tumor necrosis factor therapy. Arch Dermatol 2008;144: 1360–6.

115. Outland JD, Keiran SJ, Schikler KN, et al. Multicentric reticulohistiocytosis in a 14-year-old girl. Pediatr Dermatol 2002;19:527–31.

116. Valencia IC, Colsky A, Berman B. Multicentric reticulohistiocytosis associated with recurrent breast carcinoma. J Am Acad Dermatol 1998;39:864–6.

117. Ponti G, Ponz de Leon M. Muir-Torre syndrome. Lancet Oncol 2005;6:980–7.

118. Cohen PR, Kohn SR, Kurzrock R. Association of sebaceous gland tumors and internal malignancy: the Muir-Torre syndrome. Am J Med 1991;90:606–13.

119. Schwartz RA, Torre DP. The Muir-Torre syndrome: a 25-year retrospect. J Am Acad Dermatol 1995;33:90–104.

120. Mangold E, Rahner N, Friedrichs N, et al. MSH6 mutation in Muir-Torre syndrome: could this be a rare finding? Br J Dermatol 2007;156:158–62.

121. Boland CR, Thibodeau SN, Hamilton SR, et al. A National Cancer Institute Workshop on Microsatellite Instability for cancer detection and familial predisposition: development of international criteria for the determination of microsatellite instability in colorectal cancer. Cancer Res 1998;58:5248–57.

122. Rapini RR. Practical dermatopathology. St. Louis: Elsevier Mosby; 2005.

123. Lee D, Grossman M, Schneiderman P, et al. Genetics of skin appendage neoplasms and related syndromes. J Med Genet 2005;42:811–9.

124. Fernandezherrera J, Pedraz J. Necrobiotic xanthogranuloma. Semin Cutan Med Surg 2007;26:108–13.

125. Finan MC, Winkelmann RK. Necrobiotic xanthogranuloma with paraproteinemia. a review of 22 cases. Medicine (Baltimore) 1986;65:376–88.

126. Ugurlu S, Bartley GB, Gibson LE. Necrobiotic xanthogranuloma: long-term outcome of ocular and systemic involvement. Am J Ophthalmol 2000;129:651–7.

127. Mehregan DA, Winkelmann RK. Necrobiotic xanthogranuloma. Arch Dermatol 1992;128:94–100.

128. Fortson JS, Schroeter AL. Necrobiotic xanthogranuloma with IgA paraproteinemia and extracutaneous involvement. Am J Dermatopathol 1990;12:579–84.

129. Venencie PY, Puissant A, Verola O, et al. Necrobiotic xanthogranuloma with myeloma. a case report. Cancer 1987;59:588–92.

130. Oumeish OY, Oumeish I, Tarawneh M, et al. Necrobiotic xanthogranuloma associated with paraproteinemia and non-Hodgkin's lymphoma developing

into chronic lymphocytic leukemia: the first case reported in the literature and review of the literature. Int J Dermatol 2006;45:306–10.

131. Lookingbill DP, Spangler N, Helm KF. Cutaneous metastases in patients with metastatic carcinoma: a retrospective study of 4020 patients. J Am Acad Dermatol 1993;29:228–36.

132. Lookingbill DP, Spangler N, Sexton FM. Skin involvement as the presenting sign of internal carcinoma. A retrospective study of 7316 cancer patients. J Am Acad Dermatol 1990;22:19–26.

133. Saeed S, Keehn CA, Morgan MB. Cutaneous metastasis: a clinical, pathological, and immunohistochemical appraisal. J Cutan Pathol 2004;31:419–30.

134. Schwartz RA. Cutaneous metastatic disease. J Am Acad Dermatol 1995;33: 161–82 [quiz 183–6].

135. Sariya D, Ruth K, Adams-McDonnell R, et al. Clinicopathologic correlation of cutaneous metastases: experience from a cancer center. Arch Dermatol 2007; 143:613–20.

136. Schwartz RA. Histopathologic aspects of cutaneous metastatic disease. J Am Acad Dermatol 1995;33:649–57.

Chronic Venous Disease

Claire D. Wolinsky, BA[a,c], Heidi Waldorf, MD[b,c,*]

KEYWORDS
- Venous disease • Vasculitis • Venous ulcer • Varicose veins
- Thrombophlebitis

Venous diseases often present with characteristic cutaneous manifestations. The importance of diagnosing and treating dermatologic findings of chronic venous disease should be emphasized, because the estimated prevalence is as high as 17% in men and 40% in women.[1] Varicose veins, which are one skin finding, are linked to chronic venous insufficiency and to the associated acute venous diseases, superficial thrombophlebitis and deep vein thrombosis. Several other cutaneous features are unique to acute or chronic diseases and should be recognized. Appropriate management of these disorders is necessary to avoid progression of disease and potential complications.

A separate category of venous disease is vasculitis. When targeted at the veins, vasculitis is labeled *cutaneous necrotizing venous vasculitis*. The shared skin finding in this group of disorders is purpura. The appearance of purpura may be diagnostic of a primary idiopathic disease or may help diagnose an underlying systemic disorder. The pattern of purpura should be differentiated from the other purpuric dermatoses, which differ in pathogenesis and management.

ACUTE VENOUS DISEASE
Superficial Venous Phlebitis and Thrombosis

Superficial phlebitis is the inflammation of a superficial vein that may be associated with the presence of a thrombus or may exist independently. A palpable cord in the area of thrombophlebitis is the classic cutaneous sign and can present with the characteristic clinical symptoms of warmth, pain, and erythema.[2–5]

Epidemiology and etiology

Superficial thrombophlebitis (STP) is most commonly seen in women. The mean age of onset is approximately 60 years old.[2] Varicose veins are the most frequently associated finding in patients who have STP, although it is caused by other entities, such as those listed in **Box 1**. In normal veins, catheters and needles may induce trauma or introduce bacteria and may lead to superficial phlebitis, STP, or superficial septic

[a] Albany Medical College, 47 New Scotland Avenue, Albany, NY 12208, USA
[b] The Mount Sinai Center Department of Dermatology, 5 East 98th Street, 5th Floor, New York, NY 10029, USA
[c] Department of Dermatology, The Mount Sinai School of Medicine, New York, NY 10029, USA
* Corresponding author.
E-mail address: hwaldorf@earthlink.net (H. Waldorf).

Med Clin N Am 93 (2009) 1333–1346
doi:10.1016/j.mcna.2009.08.001
0025-7125/09/$ – see front matter © 2009 Elsevier Inc. All rights reserved.

Box 1
Causes of superficial thrombophlebitis[3–5]

Varicose veins

Drugs

    Potassium chloride

    Diazepam

    Antibiotics

    Oral contraceptives

Infection

    Klebsiella

    Staphylococcus aureus

    Enterobacter

    Proteus[5]

Malignancy

Hypercoagulable states

Immunologic disorders

    Buerger's disease

    Behçet's disease

    Systemic lupus

    Collagen diseases

---

thrombophlebitis.[3] Drugs also may cause superficial phlebitis. Additionally, STP is seen as a finding in patients who have thrombophilia, Behçet's disease, and Buerger disease. When an associated underlying malignancy is present, a migratory phlebitis, known as Trousseau's sign, is characteristic.

STP of the chest wall, referred to as Mondor's disease, can be caused by trauma, excessive physical activity, breast surgery, inflammatory conditions, infection, mastitis, breast abscess, or pendulous breasts. Among cases of Mondor's disease, 12% will be associated with breast carcinoma.[6] In men, Mondor's may affect the dorsal penile vein. In these patients, sexual activity is a predisposing factor when it occurs 24 to 48 hours before the development of thrombophlebitis.[3]

Risk factors

Obesity, substitutive hormonal therapy, oral contraceptives, and a history of thromboembolism are risk factors for STP.[2] General risk factors for thrombosis, such as recent trauma or surgery and prolonged immobilization, also place patients at risk for STP because of endothelial damage or venous stasis.

Pathogenesis

In STP, a neutrophilic-predominant inflammatory cellular infiltrate is seen at the large and medium-sized veins of the upper subcutis and lower dermis. Vessel wall thickening occurs from edema and exudation of inflammatory cells. Later, the lesion may include lymphocytes and histiocytes, and connective tissue proliferation results in the formation of a palpable cord. Occlusion of the lumen of the vein by thrombi eventually undergoes recanalization over 2 weeks to 6 months.[3]

Skin findings

Varicose veins Varicose veins are tortuous, superficial veins of the leg that result from dysfunctional valves (**Fig. 1**). Typically, they are located at the medial region of the calf. Patients may report an associated aching or heaviness, itching, or swelling. Acutely, complications of varicose veins are cellulitis and STP.[7] Over time, more features of chronic venous disease may arise. In the damaged varicose veins of the lower leg is where 70% of STP cases develop.[2]

Palpable cord STP manifests as an erythematous nodule or cord that may be tender, hot, or painful. Because the most common site of origin is varicose veins, STP is most frequently noted on the lower legs. The cord will resolve in 2 weeks when not associated with an underlying disease. Postinflammatory hyperpigmentation may remain.[3]

The same finding of an indurated cord is seen from the breast to the axilla region in Mondor's disease. Unlike STP of the legs, the cord may persist for weeks to months, although the pain usually resolves after several days. A unique finding is the puckering of skin noted as the inflammation resolves.[4,6]

Diagnosis

Clinical diagnosis of STP is usually sufficient, however, Duplex ultrasonography may be performed in patients at risk to rule out concurrent deep vein thrombosis.[4] When STP is recurrent, migratory, or more widespread, or it occurs without the presence of varicose veins, screening should be performed to identify a systemic disease or an underlying malignancy.[5] In patients who have a history of instrumentation of the venous system or if they require a differential from cellulitis, a Gram stain and culture may help identify a causative pathogen.

Treatment

Besides being painful, STP is believed to be a benign condition unless accompanied by a deep venous thrombosis (DVT). Symptomatic treatment can be treated with compression stockings and oral nonsteroidal anti-inflammatory drugs (NSAIDs) as needed. Topical analgesics used locally also have shown benefit. If topical analgesics are not tolerated, topical heparin has been shown to shorten the duration of signs and symptoms.[5] In general, patients should be urged to avoid bed rest, which may predispose them to DVT.

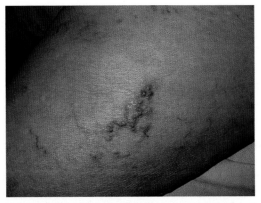

Fig. 1. Varicosities. Early cutaneous manifestations of venous valve dysfunction include tortuous, superficial veins of the lower extremities. (*Courtesy of* Jacob Levitt, MD, New York, NY.)

Prophylaxis with low molecular weight heparin is not routinely necessary, because STP alone has not been proven to be a predisposing risk factor for venous thromboembolism. Prophylaxis may be necessary for patients at high risk for developing a DVT or when the thrombus is located less than 1 cm from the saphenous–femoral junction.[3]

CHRONIC VENOUS DISEASE
Chronic Venous Insufficiency

Chronic venous insufficiency (CVI) is a condition caused by venous hypertension, resulting most commonly from dysfunctional valves in the veins of the lower extremities. Several cutaneous manifestations are characteristic of the disease.

Epidemiology and etiology

The two main causes of CVI are varicose veins and postphlebotic syndrome.[8] Approximately half of patients who have varicose veins have a positive family history. Varicose veins are three times more common in women than men and has a peak incidence of onset between ages 30 and 40 years.[4]

Risk factors

Recognized risk factors for CVI include those implicated in the development of varicose veins or venous thrombosis. The associated risks are prolonged standing, obesity, pregnancy, surgery, trauma, malignancy, female gender, and genetics.[9]

Pathogenesis

In the pathogenesis of varicose veins, incompetent one-way valves of the deep veins in the leg fail to maintain a unidirectional flow of venous blood. When the calf muscle contracts, the veins are compressed, but backflow leads to pooling of blood and hypertension in the superficial veins and capillaries of the skin. Over time, the high pressure in the vessels of the skin leads to soft tissue damage and inflammation. The resultant swollen and leaky endothelial cells allow for the extravasation of fibrinogen, which is responsible for the development of pericapillary fibrin cuffs.[9–11]

The insult in CVI is cyclical, with each step leading to further stasis and increasing venous pressure. Venous stasis leads to fibrosis and lipodermatosclerosis, which promotes thrombosis.[4] As CVI progresses, the delivery of nutrients to the skin is further obstructed, manifesting in tissue breakdown and ulcerations.

Cutaneous findings

Edema The first noticeable change is dependent, pitting edema in the medial region of the lower legs and ankles.[10] Edema eventually extends to the entire distal third of the leg. Legs may be tender to palpation. Patients complain of aching and a sense of heaviness in their legs that is exacerbated by prolonged standing and improved by lying down.[9,10]

Stasis dermatitis At any stage in CVI, an eczematous dermatitis may present with findings of erythematous, papular, scaling, oozing, or crusting lesions found at the medial supramalleolar region. Over time, hyperpigmentation becomes more prominent secondary to chronic erythrocyte extravasation, with subsequent hemosiderin deposit (**Fig. 2**). Petechiae may be present in combination with evidence of old hemorrhages.[9–12]

Because of the pruritic nature of stasis dermatitis, excoriations may be present. Chronic scratching of the skin leads to lichenification.[4] Excoriations also provide an open portal for bacteria. Topical antibiotics or any of the various topical agents used by patients to treat dryness or scaling can lead to contact dermatitis. The

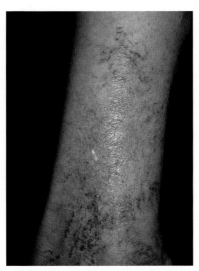

Fig. 2. Stasis dermatitis. In the presence of lower leg varicosities, further soft tissue injury leads to the extravasation of red blood vessels. Hemosiderosis results and may accompany clinical symptoms of dermatitis, such as pruritus. (*Courtesy of* Jacob Levitt, MD, New York, NY.)

appearance of vesicles is more common with contact dermatitis and may help in the differential. A generalized distribution is also more characteristic of contact dermatitis than of stasis dermatitis. Further complicating the clinical picture, irritant dermatitis may also be superimposed in the presence of secretions from exudative ulcers.[12]

Atrophie blanche In CVI, small porcelain white plaques, known as atrophie blanche, may be noted within areas of stasis dermatitis. The atrophic stellate lesions have characteristic irregular edges with a hyperpigmentated border. Telangiectasias are typically seen at the periphery of the plaques. Painful, purpuric, small punched-out ulcers may also be present and are difficult to treat. Almost all patients who have atrophie blanche show signs of venous insufficiency.[11] When not associated with stasis dermatitis, atrophie blanche may be the result of an underlying coagulopathy or autoimmune disease. The term *idiopathic livedoid vasculopathy* is used when atrophie blanche presents as its own entity.[13]

Lipodermatosclerosis Lipodermatosclerosis, a later finding in CVI, is the result of inflammation, followed by fibrosis replacing subcutaneous fat. This skin finding manifests as an indurated plaque first noticed at the medial ankle. Eventually, circumferential extension of the sclerotic area in the lower third of the leg impedes venous and lymphatic flow (**Fig. 3**). The appearance of the pigmented, strangulated site of fibrosis with edema above and below has been termed *inverted champagne bottle* or *piano leg*. The "groove sign" is formed when varicose veins are found within the region of sclerosis. Chronic lymphedema of the leg can also result from the fibrotic blockage.[10] When lipodermatosclerosis is found with verrucous changes and cutaneous hypertrophy, the condition is known as *elephantiasis nostras verrucous*.[4]

Lipodermatosclerosis leads to limitations of movement and pain in the afflicted ankles. Patients become more sedentary and CVI is further exacerbated.

Venous ulcers Mostly found around the medial supramalleolar region, venous ulcers are shallow and irregular (**Fig. 4**). Venous ulcers are typically larger and may be less painful

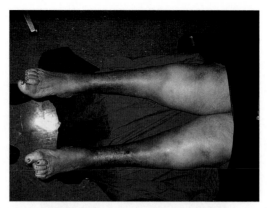

Fig. 3. Lipodermatosclerosis. Bilateral lower leg induration and erythema is seen in the lower third of the legs. The edema above and below the scarring give the appearance of a "champagne bottle." (*Courtesy of* Jacob Levitt, MD, New York, NY.)

than nonvenous ulcers. The base of the lesion is red and necrotic and the borders are sloped. Yellow exudate is usually present.[8] Because venous ulcers are a late finding of CVI, patients typically have other skin findings, such as varicose veins, lipodermatosclerosis, lymphedema, pigmentation, atrophie blanche, and stasis dermatitis. Damage to the valves in venous insufficiency is permanent. Therefore, CVI is a lifelong disorder, and venous ulcers tend to recur in as high as 70% of treated patients.[10]

Squamous cell carcinoma may arise in nonhealing venous ulcers. Changes in the features or symptoms of an ulcer may indicate malignant transformation.[9]

Acroangiodermatitis (of Mali) Referred to as pseudo-Kaposi's sarcoma, acroangiodermatitis typically presents as purple nodules, macules, patches, or plaques found on the dorsal aspect of the foot, the toes, and the extensor surface of the distal lower

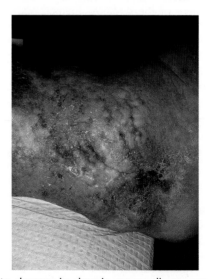

Fig. 4. Venous ulcer. Late changes in chronic venous disease are witnessed by irregular, shallow ulcers seen here in the lateral malleolar region in the context of elephantitis. (*Courtesy of* Jacob Levitt, MD, New York, NY.)

extremities. The lesions may enlarge, ulcerate, or become painful over time. Other cutaneous features of CVI are usually present when acroangiodermatitis is seen. Less commonly, acroangiodermatitis is associated with arteriovenous malformations.[9,10]

Diagnosis

CVI can be diagnosed based solely on clinical findings. If evaluation of venous anatomy and physiology is needed, color duplex ultrasound is considered the gold standard.[11] Additionally, the severity of venous reflux can be evaluated using photoplethysmography and air plethysmography. When a venous ulcer must be differentiated from an arterial ulcer, Doppler ultrasound may be used to measure the ankle–brachial index (ABI) to detect arterial insufficiency.[9] If the ABI is normal, an arterial origin for the ulcer may likely be ruled out.

Treatment

Venous insufficiency is chronic and many of the treatments are aimed at preventing advanced manifestations of the disease. Because the disease is exacerbated by obesity and prolonged standing, weight loss and leg elevation are beneficial. Lower leg stockings, bandages, and pneumatic compression can provide mechanical support for venous return. Pressure on the lower legs restricts backflow from damaged valves and limits pooling and stasis of blood. Use of these garments also can protect against trauma to the limb.[10,11]

Compression stockings are classified into four categories based on the extent of compression at the ankle.[11] The recommended compression stocking ankle pressure for CVI is 35 to 40 mmHg and may be increased to 60 mmHg when disease is severe. Best results are achieved when garments are worn immediately on rising from bed and are applied daily.[10] Alternatively, a rigid inelastic bandage, such as the traditional Unna boot, which is a moist zinc-impregnated paste bandage that is applied and allowed to dry, can be used short-term in patients who are ambulatory but unable to wear compression stockings.[11]

Surgery has also been used to treat varicose veins and may be beneficial in the management of CVI. Options include endovascular surgery, sclerotherapy, radiofrequency ablation, and endovenous laser therapy. In endovascular surgery, incompetent saphenous veins are identified by ultrasound, ligated and cut, and stripped.[9] Sclerotherapy involves the direct administration of a sclerosing agent to the identified incompetent vein, followed by compression for several weeks. The newer minimally invasive endovascular techniques use radiofrequency or laser thermal heating to occlude incompetent saphenous veins, with more rapid recovery and fewer complications than standard ligation and stripping for appropriate patients.[10,14]

Other treatments are directed at specific cutaneous manifestations of CVI. Stasis dermatitis may be treated with emollients and short-term mid-potent steroid ointment. In the acute exudative stage, wet dressings can be beneficial and a corticosteroid cream is preferred over an ointment.[10] Pain associated with atrophie blanche can be treated with intralesional triamcinolone injections.[4] Steroids, however, should not be used on venous ulcers because concerns about further skin breakdown and increased risk for infection.

Venous ulcer therapy includes debridement of necrotic tissue, either chemical or mechanical, to allow for reepithelialization and adequate healing. Devitalized tissue also must be removed to reduce the risk for infection. Various types of specialized occlusive dressings are also used to maintain a moist environment, which helps dissolve necrotic debris and accelerate healing. These dressings include absorptive hydrocolloid bandages and pastes and newer preparations involving growth factors.[15]

Because CVI patients have a higher risk for contact dermatitis, topical antibiotic preparations should be used with caution.[11]

In general, patients should also be screened for anemia and instructed to maintain a nutritious diet to ensure proper healing. Medical therapy, such as aspirin and pentoxifylline, has been suggested for treating healing venous ulcers, although the benefit is still unclear.[10] Although most venous ulcers are colonized with bacteria, antibiotics are not administered routinely.[11] Deep biopsies should be taken routinely in suspicious, nonhealing ulcers to evaluate for squamous cell carcinoma. Skin grafting, with either autologous or bioengineered skin substitutes, can also be considered in nonhealing ulcers that are not responsive to other treatments.[11,16]

CUTANEOUS VASCULITIS AND OTHER PURPURIC SYNDROMES
Cutaneous Small Vessel Vasculitis

Cutaneous small vessel vasculitis (CSVV) is defined by immunologic or inflammatory-induced damage of the postcapillary venules localized to the skin. The typical clinical manifestation is erythematous, nonblanching papules called *palpable purpura*. Other names for CSVV include cutaneous leukoclastic vasculitis, cutaneous necrotizing venulitis, and hypersensitivity vasculitis.[17–20]

Etiology and epidemiology
CSVV may arise in the absence of an underlying systemic disease at a mean age of onset between 34 nd 49 years of age.[17] Women are two- to threefold more likely to develop CSVV than men. Specific variants of CSVV that present with characteristic clinical symptoms and findings affect a more defined population group. For example, Henoch-Schönlein purpura (HSP) and acute hemorrhagic edema of childhood are seen in age groups younger than 10 and 2 years, respectively.[17,18]

Most commonly, patients present with idiopathic primary CSVV (30%–60%) involving only the skin.[18] CSVV may be triggered by precipitating infections (22%) or drug hypersensitivities (20%), or may be the manifestation of a malignancy (<5%).[20] Additionally, several systemic inflammatory disorders are associated with CSVV, such as those listed in **Box 2**.

Exacerbating factors
Primary CSVV may be exacerbated by exercise, extreme temperatures, sun exposures, and prolonged stasis.[19]

Pathogenesis
Immune complexes have been implicated in the pathogenesis of CSVV. The proposed series of events begins with the deposition of immune complexes at the wall of postcapillary venules, followed by activation of the complement system. The subsequent release of chemokines mainly attracts neutrophils, along with a mix of monocytes and lymphocytes. The proposed pathogenesis is supported by the characteristic histology of CSVV with a neutrophilic-predominant cellular infiltrate and fibrinoid necrosis of blood vessel walls. The inflammatory cells are believed to release several factors that lead to increased permeability of the blood vessel wall and endothelial swelling, ultimately ending in fibrosis and necrosis of the wall.[17–20]

Box 2
Causes of cutaneous small vessel vasculitis[18–20]

Chronic disorders

    Connective tissue disease

        Rheumatoid arthritis

        Behçet's disease

        Sjögren syndrome

        Systemic lupus erythematous

    Vasculitis

    Inflammatory bowel disease

    Cryoglobulinemia

Malignancy

Drug reactions

    Beta-lactams

    Sulfa drugs

    Penicillin

    Nonsteroidal anti-inflammatory drugs

Infections

    Bacterial

        Streptococcus

        Staphylococcus

        Clamydia

        Mycobacterium

    Viral

        Hepatitis B or C/HIV

    Fungal

        Candida

Skin findings of cutaneous small vessel vasculitis

Palpable purpura Damage to the venule wall allows extravasation of red blood cells into the adjacent dermis, which manifests clinically as purpura. Purpura in CSVV is typically localized to the dependent areas of the body and most commonly to the lower legs (**Fig. 5**). Early on the lesion is macular, but over time the purpura becomes papular. Progression to plaques, vesicles, and pustules may occur. In primary CSVV, ulceration, nodules, bullae, and necrosis are seen less frequently than in other forms of CSVV.[19] Over 1 to 4 weeks, individual crops of purpura commonly resolve.[18] Areas of postinflammatory hyperpigmentation may be seen with resolution of the disease or alongside more acute lesions.

Purpura may have associated symptoms, including pruritus, pain, stinging, or burning. Systemic symptoms such as fever, malaise, arthralgias, myalgias, and anorexia may arise with the onset of CSVV. Extracutaneous organ involvement suggest the presence of a systemic vasculitis.[20]

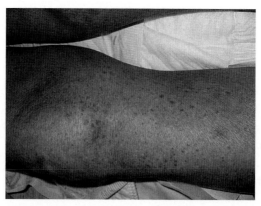

Fig. 5. Palpable purpura. Petechiae on the lower extremities are characteristic of cutaneous small vessel vasculitis. (*Courtesy of* Jacob Levitt, MD, New York, NY.)

Skin findings specific to subgroups

Acute hemorrhagic edema of childhood Acute hemorrhagic edema of childhood (AHEC) is a disease that may be idiopathic but is more frequently associated with a triggering drug or infection. Facial edema may be the initial presentation, followed by petechial and ecchymotic lesions involving the face and distal extremities. Target-like purpuric lesions may also develop regions of bullae or necrosis. Pain may be an associated symptom. The disease is self-limiting and lasts between 1 and 3 weeks.[17,18]

AHEC has been categorized under HSP; however, unlike HSP, it is associated with no extracutaneous findings. In addition to the palpable purpura found on the back, buttock, and extensor region of the lower extremities, HSP vasculitis afflicts the gastrointestinal and renal systems. Systemic features, such as arthritis and arthralgia, are also common in HSP.[18,19]

Urticarial vasculitis The normocomplement subtype of urticarial vasculitis (UV) is typically limited to cutaneous involvement, whereas the hypocomplement group of UV most often leads to systemic features in addition to the typical skin findings.

The cutaneous manifestations of both types of UV are recurrent or chronic urticarial lesions with or without purpuric foci. Unlike typical urticaria, erythematous, indurated wheals of UV may not resolve within 24 hours and may result in residual pigmentation. The urticaria may be pruritic, painful, or burning. Other skin findings of UV are angioedema, livedo reticularis, nodules, and bullae.[17–19]

Essential mixed cryoglobulinemia Essential mixed cryoglobulinemia (EMC) may present as a systemic disease or be limited to the skin. Palpable purpura appearing in the dependent areas of the lower extremities is the characteristic cutaneous feature. The nonpruritic or painful lesions appear episodically and last between 3 and 10 days.[17] Triggers are cold temperatures or prolonged sitting or standing. Livedo reticularis, urticaria, digital ulceration, and gangrene are also seen in EMC.[17,19]

Diagnosis

A thorough history and physical should ideally identify precipitating drugs, infections, or an underlying chronic disease as the cause of CSVV. A cutaneous biopsy is diagnostic and should be performed in a lesion between 18 and 48 hours after it arises.[19] Because primary CSVV is a diagnosis of exclusion, further workup may include appropriate laboratory screening, such as listed in **Box 3**. Frequently, the erythrocyte sediment is elevated in patients who have CSVV.[18]

Treatment

CSVV is self-limited and typically occurs in patients as a single episode. Therefore, treating symptoms may be all that is warranted. Bed rest, leg elevation, compression stocking, antihistamines, and NSAIDs can help relieve pruritus and pain. Colchicine and dapsone have also been used therapeutically, but results do not show a consistent benefit.[17–20] When CSVV is severely symptomatic, recurrent, or progressive, or presents with nodular, ulcerating, or vesicular purpura, oral corticosteroids are indicated. Prednisone may be given at 0.5 to 1 mg/kg daily and tapered over a prolonged period to prevent rebound.[19] Steroid-sparing agents, such as azathioprine and cyclosporine, may be useful in treating patients who have more chronic CSVV.

Purpuric Syndromes

Pigmented purpuric dermatoses

Pigmented purpuric dermatoses (PPD) are believed to result from capillaritis characterized by pinpoint brown-red macules representing red blood cell extravasation and hemosiderin deposit.

Etiology and epidemiology PPD affects men more frequently than women and most common occurs between ages 30 and 60 years.[21] More specifically, Schamberg's disease, a PPD subtype, affects mostly older men. Other subcategories, Lichen aureus and Majocchi's disease, appear most often in young adulthood, and Gougerot-Blum syndrome typically presents between ages 40 and 60 years.[6,22]

The cause of PPD is unknown. Nonetheless, certain drugs may be triggering factors. The typical presentation of PPD is insidious, but when caused by an inciting factor, onset is rapid. Exercise, contact allergies, and alcohol ingestion also have been

---

Box 3
Laboratory screening for cause of cutaneous small vessel vasculitis[18,19]

Initial laboratories

    Complete blood cell count with differential

    Erythrocyte sediment

    Urinalysis

    Complete metabolic panel (includes creatinine and liver function testing)

    Infectious serologies/culture

    Hepatitis B and C serologies

More specific evaluations

    Cryoglobulins

    Complement (CH50, C3, C4)

    Antinuclear antibody

    Rheumatoid factor

    Serum protein electrophoresis

    Antineutrophil cytoplasmic antibodies

proposed as causes for the disease. Some systemic diseases are associated with PPD, such as diabetes mellitus, rheumatoid arthritis, lupus erythematous, thyroid dysfunction, hereditary spherocytosis, hematologic disorders, hepatic disease, porphyria, malignancies, and hyperlipidemia.[22]

Pathogenesis The typical histologic picture of PPD is inflammation of the superficial blood vessels of the dermis with endothelial swelling, erythrocyte extravasation, and the presence of a perivascular lymphocytic infiltrate and hemosiderin-laden macrophages. Unlike vasculitis, no fibrosis of the vessels occurs.[6,21,22]

Skin findings

Pinpoint hemorrhages (purpura) Pinpoint, nonblanching hemorrhages resembling cayenne pepper appear mostly bilaterally at the lower legs. Acutely, the lesions are red, but with age they become a brown-rust color (**Fig. 6**). In some variants, a golden or tan hue is noted. A cluster of macules may take months to years to resolve and usually recurs. The discrete macules may become confluent and form patches and plaques. Pinpoint hemorrhages may be pruritic or asymptomatic.[21,22]

Telangiectasias Telangiectasias are described in Majocchi's disease. Annular bluish-red macules with dark-red telangiectasias on the lower legs are the unique feature of Majocchi's. The telangiectasias are typically located at the border of lesions, along with cayenne-pepper petechiae.[6,21,22]

Lichenoid papules Small flat-topped elevated papules occur along with pinpoint hemorrhages on the lower legs in Lichen aureus disease and Gougerot-Blum syndrome.[22]

Diagnosis and treatment PPD may be diagnosed based on the clinical picture. When the diagnosis is not straightforward, laboratory screening to rule out a thrombocytopenia or coagulation disorder is reasonable. A biopsy may also be performed if the differential diagnosis is unclear. The presence of extracutaneous symptoms warrants a more complete review of blood work to rule out an underlying systemic disease.

No treatment has proven to be effective. Super-potent topical steroids may be used for 4 to 6 weeks to allow for an adequate therapeutic trial. Patients who have pruritus experience most benefit from using steroids.[22]

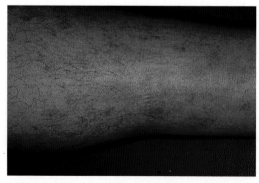

Fig. 6. Pinpoint hemorrhages. Cayenne-pepper papules seen here on the lower leg of a man who presented with Schamberg's purpura. (*Courtesy of* Mark Lebwohl, MD, New York, NY.)

SUMMARY

Identifying characteristic cutaneous findings is important in determining the appropriate management of certain venous diseases. The health care provider should be familiar with the classic description of patterns and distributions of skin manifestations, such as varicose veins, stasis dermatitis, palpable cord, petechiae, and telangiectasias. In addition to the gross appearance of the skin, a skin biopsy may help elucidate a diagnosis. General treatment and prevention of the underlying venous pathology is essential. Furthermore, specific management of skin findings should include therapy to ameliorate progression of disease and symptomatology when warranted.

REFERENCES

1. Robertson L, Evans C, Fowkes FGR. Epidemiology of chronic venous disease. Phlebology 2008;23:103–11.
2. Decousus H, Magali E, Guillot K, et al. Superficial vein thrombosis: risk factors, diagnosis, and treatment. Curr Opin Pulm Med 2003;9(5):393–7.
3. Rodriguez-Peralto JL, Carrillo R, Rosales B, et al. Superficial thrombophlebitis. Semin Cutan Med Surg 2007;26:71–6.
4. Wolff K, Johnson RA, Section 16. Skin signs of vascular insufficiency. In: Wolff K, Johnson RA, editors. Fitzpatrick's color atlas and synopsis of clinical dermatology. 6th edition. Available at: http://www.accessmedicine.com/content.aspx?aID=5189520.
5. Cesarone MR, Belcaro G, Agus G, et al. Management of superficial vein thrombosis and thrombophlebitis: status and expert opinion document. Angiology 2007;58(1):7S–15S.
6. Piette W. Purpura and coagulation. In: Bolognia JL, Jorizzo JL, Rapini RP, editors, Dermatology, vol. 1. Philadelphia: Elsevier's Health Sciences; 2003. p. 355–63.
7. Fritsch P, Burgdorf W, Murphey G, et al. Skin diseases in Europe. Eur J Dermatol 2008;18(2):211–9.
8. Abbade LP, Lastoria S. Venous ulcer: epidemiology, physiopathology, diagnosis and treatment. Int Society Dermatol 2005;44:449–56.
9. Burton CS, Burkhart C, Goldsmith LA. Cutaneous changes in venous and lymphatic insufficiency. In: Wolff K, Goldsmith LA, Katz SI, et al, editors. Fitzpatrick's dermatology in general medicine. 7th edition. Available at: http://www.accessmedicine.com/content.aspx?aID=2994438.
10. Lin P, Phillips T. Ulcers. In: Bolognia JL, Jorizzo JL, Rapini RP, editors, Dermatology, vol. 2. Philadelphia: Elsevier's Health Sciences; 2003. p. 1633.
11. Valencia IC, Falabella A, Kirsner RS, et al. Chronic venous insufficiency and venous leg ulceration. J Am Acad Dermatol 2001;44:401–21.
12. Fritsch PO, Reider N. Other eczematous eruptions. In: Bolognia JL, Jorizzo JL, Rapini RP, editors, Dermatology, vol. 1. Philadelphia: Elsevier's Health Sciences; 2003. p. 219–21.
13. Jorizzo JL. Livedoid vasculopathy: what is it? Arch Dermatol 1998;134:491–3.
14. Navarro L, Min RJ, Bone C. Endovenous laser: a new minimally invasive treatment for varicose veins—preliminary observations using an 810 nm diode laser. Dermatol Surg 2001;27:117–22.
15. Harrison-Balestra C, Eaglstein WH, Falabela AF, et al. Recombinant human platelet-derived growth factor for refractory nondiabetic ulcers: a retrospective series. Dermatol Surg 2002;28(8):755–60.
16. Phillips TJ. Current approaches to venous ulcers and compression. Dermatol Surg 2001;27:611–21.

17. Hannon CW, Swerlick RA. Vasculitis. In: Bolognia JL, Jorizzo JL, Rapini RP, editors, Dermatology, vol. 1. Philadelphia: Elsevier's Health Sciences; 2003. p. 381–402.

18. Soter NA, Diaz-Perez J. Cutaneous necrotizing venulitis. In: Wolff K, Goldsmith LA, Katz SI, et al, editors. Fitzpatrick's dermatology in general medicine. 7th edition. Available at: http://www.accessmedicine.com/content.aspx?aID=2961660.

19. Russell JP, Gibson LE. Primary cutaneous small vessel vasculitis: approach to diagnosis and treatment. Int J Dermatol 2006;45:3–13.

20. Carlson JA, Chen K. Cutaneous vasculitis update: small vessel neutrophilic vasculitis syndromes. Am J Dermatopathol 2006;28(6):486–506.

21. Wolff K, Johnson RA. Section 7. Miscellaneous inflammatory disorders. In: Wolff K, Johnson RA, editors. Fitzpatrick's color atlas and synopsis of clinical dermatology. 6th edition. Available at: http://www.accessmedicine.com/content.aspx?aID=5201183.

22. Sardana K, Sarkar R, Sehgal VN. Pigmented purpuric dermatoses: an overview. Int Society of Dermatol 2004;43:482–8.

Index

Note: Page numbers of article titles are in **boldface** type.

Med Clin N Am 93 (2009) 1347–1363
doi:10.1016/S0025-7125(09)00134-5
0025-7125/09/$ – see front matter © 2009 Elsevier Inc. All rights reserved.

medical.theclinics.com

United States Postal Service

Statement of Ownership, Management, and Circulation
(All Periodicals Publications Except Requester Publications)

1. Publication Title
Medical Clinics of North America

2. Publication Number
3 3 7 - 3 4 0

3. Filing Date
9/15/09

4. Issue Frequency
Jan, Mar, May, Jul, Sep, Nov

5. Number of Issues Published Annually
6

6. Annual Subscription Price
$187.00

7. Complete Mailing Address of Known Office of Publication (Not printer) (Street, city, county, state, and ZIP+4®)
Elsevier Inc.
360 Park Avenue South
New York, NY 10010-1710

Contact Person
Stephen Bushing

Telephone (Include area code)
215-239-3688

8. Complete Mailing Address of Headquarters or General Business Office of Publisher (Not printer)
Elsevier Inc., 360 Park Avenue South, New York, NY 10010-1710

9. Full Names and Complete Mailing Addresses of Publisher, Editor, and Managing Editor (Do not leave blank)

Publisher (Name and complete mailing address)
John Schrefer, Elsevier, Inc., 1600 John F. Kennedy Blvd. Suite 1800, Philadelphia, PA 19103-2899

Editor (Name and complete mailing address)
Rachel Glover, Elsevier, Inc., 1600 John F. Kennedy Blvd. Suite 1800, Philadelphia, PA 19103-2899

Managing Editor (Name and complete mailing address)
Catherine Bewick, Elsevier, Inc., 1600 John F. Kennedy Blvd. Suite 1800, Philadelphia, PA 19103-2899

10. Owner (Do not leave blank. If the publication is owned by a corporation, give the name and address of the corporation immediately followed by the names and addresses of all stockholders owning or holding 1 percent or more of the total amount of stock. If not owned by a corporation, give the names and addresses of the individual owners. If owned by a partnership or other unincorporated firm, give its name and address as well as those of each individual owner. If the publication is published by a nonprofit organization, give its name and address.)

Full Name	Complete Mailing Address
Wholly owned subsidiary of	4520 East-West Highway
Reed/Elsevier, US holdings	Bethesda, MD 20814

11. Known Bondholders, Mortgagees, and Other Security Holders Owning or Holding 1 Percent or More of Total Amount of Bonds, Mortgages, or Other Securities. If none, check box ☐ None

Full Name	Complete Mailing Address
N/A	

12. Tax Status (For completion by nonprofit organizations authorized to mail at nonprofit rates) (Check one)
The purpose, function, and nonprofit status of this organization and the exempt status for federal income tax purposes:
☐ Has Not Changed During Preceding 12 Months
☐ Has Changed During Preceding 12 Months (Publisher must submit explanation of change with this statement)

PS Form **3526**, September 2007 (Page 1 of 3 (Instructions Page 3)) PSN 7530-01-000-9931 PRIVACY NOTICE: See our Privacy policy in www.usps.com

---

13. Publication Title
Medical Clinics of North America

14. Issue Date for Circulation Data Below
September 2009

15. Extent and Nature of Circulation

		Average No. Copies Each Issue During Preceding 12 Months	No. Copies of Single Issue Published Nearest to Filing Date
a. Total Number of Copies (Net press run)		4226	4000
b. Paid Circulation (By Mail and Outside the Mail)	(1) Mailed Outside-County Paid Subscriptions Stated on PS Form 3541. (Include paid distribution above nominal rate, advertiser's proof copies, and exchange copies)	1901	1809
	(2) Mailed In-County Paid Subscriptions Stated on PS Form 3541 (Include paid distribution above nominal rate, advertiser's proof copies, and exchange copies)		
	(3) Paid Distribution Outside the Mails Including Sales Through Dealers and Carriers, Street Vendors, Counter Sales, and Other Paid Distribution Outside USPS®	1040	1135
	(4) Paid Distribution by Other Classes Mailed Through the USPS (e.g. First-Class Mail®)		
c. Total Paid Distribution (Sum of 15b (1), (2), (3), and (4))	▲	2941	2944
d. Free or Nominal Rate Distribution (By Mail and Outside the Mail)	(1) Free or Nominal Rate Outside-County Copies Included on PS Form 3541	133	123
	(2) Free or Nominal Rate In-County Copies Included on PS Form 3541		
	(3) Free or Nominal Rate Copies Mailed at Other Classes Through the USPS (e.g. First-Class Mail)		
	(4) Free or Nominal Rate Distribution Outside the Mail (Carriers or other means)		
e. Total Free or Nominal Rate Distribution (Sum of 15d (1), (2), (3) and (4))	▲	133	123
f. Total Distribution (Sum of 15c and 15e)	▲	3074	3067
g. Copies not Distributed (See instructions to publishers #4 (page #3))	▲	1152	933
h. Total (Sum of 15f and g)	▲	4226	4000
i. Percent Paid (15c divided by 15f times 100)		95.67%	95.99%

16. Publication of Statement of Ownership
If the publication is a general publication, publication of this statement is required. Will be printed in the **November 2009** issue of this publication. ☐ Publication not required.

17. Signature and Title of Editor, Publisher, Business Manager, or Owner

[signature] Stephen R. Bushing – Subscription Services Coordinator

Date September 15, 2009

I certify that all information furnished on this form is true and complete. I understand that anyone who furnishes false or misleading information on this form or who omits material or information requested on the form may be subject to criminal sanctions (including fines and imprisonment) and/or civil sanctions (including civil penalties).

PS Form 3526, September 2007 (Page 2 of 3)

Moving?

Make sure your subscription moves with you!

To notify us of your new address, find your **Clinics Account Number** (located on your mailing label above your name), and contact customer service at:

Email: journalscustomerservice-usa@elsevier.com

800-654-2452 (subscribers in the U.S. & Canada)
314-447-8871 (subscribers outside of the U.S. & Canada)

Fax number: 314-447-8029

Elsevier Health Sciences Division
Subscription Customer Service
3251 Riverport Lane
Maryland Heights, MO 63043

*To ensure uninterrupted delivery of your subscription, please notify us at least 4 weeks in advance of move.

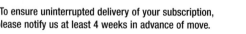